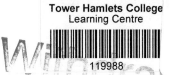

This book is to be returned on or before

the book of
ayurveda

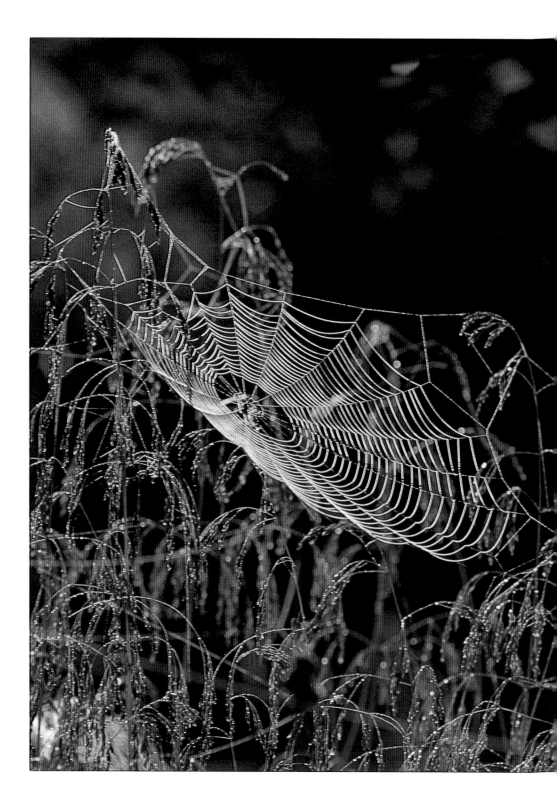

the book of ayurveda

an interactive
guide to using
Indian healing for
personal wellbeing

Judith H. Morrison

Gaia Books Limited

A GAIA ORIGINAL

Books from Gaia celebrate the vision of Gaia, the self-sustaining living Earth, and seek to help their readers live in greater personal and planetary harmony.

Editorial	Pip Morgan, Fiona Trent, Eleanor Lines
Design	Sara Mathews
Illustration	Tilney Kirkbride
Direction	Joss Pearson Patrick Nugent

To
A.D.M.

"Words do not create facts, they either describe them or distort them. The fact is always non-verbal." Sri Nisgadatta Maharaj in *I am That*.

It is my sincere hope that through this book you will glimpse the depth, beauty, and potential of Ayurveda. I apologize for any distortion of the teachings due to my interpretation and trust that in pursuing your interest in Ayurveda you will use your discrimination to find genuine and compassionate teachers.

I would like to give thanks:
For the bounty of the universe which has given me many gifts, including the privilege of studying with teachers who are part of the living tradition of Ayurveda
To my parents
To my teachers, Dr. Vasant Lad and Dr. Robert Svoboda
To my brother
To all the Staff and Friends at the Ayurvedic Institute, Albuquerque, for their love, encouragement, and support
To Anne Wyatt and Hart De Fouw for the benefit of their exceptional though different skills, without which I would never have written a book
To Dr. Vasant Lad and the Ayurvedic Press for contributing the Food Guidelines
To Will Foster for his help with the Sanskrit Sutras
To Duncan Hulin of the Devon School of Yoga for his help with the exercise sequence
To Barbara and Jack Savage, Angela Hope-Murray, Richard Barton, Pauline Dunn, and Eileen Pettit for their loving support and practical help.

Judith Morrison

Contents

FOREWORD

We live in the Age of Information, an age in which we are literally being inundated with information of all kinds. But if a little knowledge can be a dangerous thing, it can also be risky to have too much, unless you have a reliable way to organize it. This is particularly true in the realm of health and disease, for today we have a bewildering array of effective but often contradictory therapies from which to choose. Though advocates of each therapy maintain the superiority of their approach, it is clear that one remedy is good for some people sometimes, but none is appropriate in all cases at all times, because all people are not the same.

It is because living beings are so diverse that Ayurveda was developed as a medical system which can be carefully tailored to individual requirements. Ayurvedic theory has been used to organize all the many types of knowledge and varieties of therapies which have developed in India over the past 5000 years or more, and can do the same for today's therapeutic techniques. Ayurveda's theories of health and disease are also sufficiently common-sensical that they can be understood by almost anyone. Ayurveda teaches self-knowledge and self-discovery; it encourages people to learn who they are, why they stay healthy and why they get sick, and how they can change their lives so that they can maximize their healthy enjoyment of living.

Because Ayurvedic wisdom is not dependent on any particular time or space, anyone from any country can benefit from Ayurveda, so long as its concepts are properly translated into the appropriate idiom. Judith Morrison, the author of this volume, has studied Ayurveda extensively at the Ayurvedic Institute in New Mexico, USA, and both Dr. Vasant Lad and I greatly appreciate her contribution to this enormous work of translation. Read what she has written, try it out in your own life, and you will have personal experience of what Ayurveda can do for you.

Dr. Robert E. Svoboda, *Ayurvedic Physician*

The Value of Ayurveda

The increasing pace of our working lives and the amount of information that is transmitted rapidly around the world is changing our lifestyles, often to the detriment of our physical, mental, and spiritual health. You can use Ayurveda to restore balance to your life by looking at the qualities you experience through your diet, work, leisure activities, and relationships – and how these interact with your unique constitution.

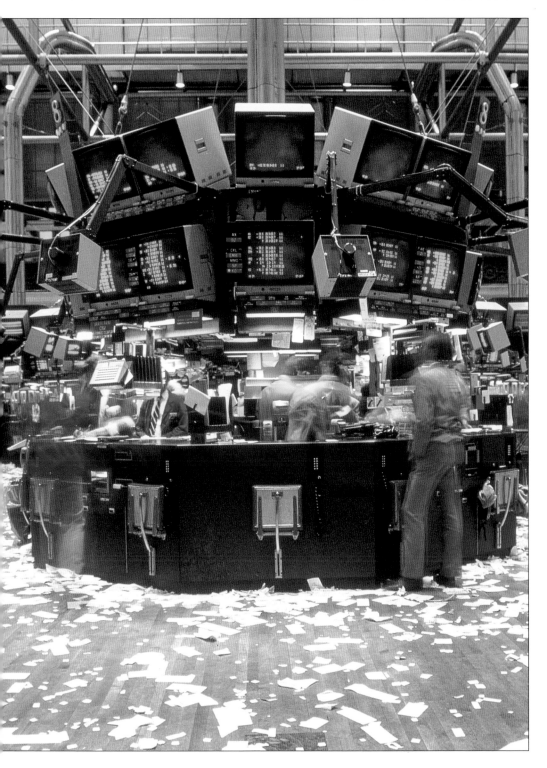

Introduction

Common knowledge tells us that a strong constitution brings good health. We all know someone whose health seems robust. Not because they keep fit, eat the right foods, and avoid excess toxins. But because they were born with a strength that equips them to cope with the stresses of modern life, and to restore an inherent equilibrium to their health. How most of us wish we could be like that: eat and do what we like, and not suffer the consequences!

But what is this constitution? Ayurveda stresses that we are all born with an individual constitution that is unique: an integral part of our being, a fixed point which is our personal baseline for health, a health equilibrium which we restore if we wish but which results in illness if we do not.

Ayurveda is a very comprehensive medical system which has been practised for generations in India as well as other countries, such as Sri Lanka. Based on the fundamental principles of life observed in deep meditations by ancient seers, Ayurveda is growing in popularity in the West. The lifestyle guidance in this book has been distilled from the vast body of Ayurvedic teachings, and is designed to help us live and eat in a way that prevents illness.

Ayurveda is a science of life which focusses on the subtle energies in all things – not only in living and inorganic things, but also in our thoughts, emotions, and actions. Each person's constitution is based on a particular relationship of three fundamental and vital energies, or doshas. Known by their Sanskrit names of vata, pitta, and kapha, these doshas are at the heart of Ayurveda. Not only do they determine your capacity for health but they also govern the way you respond to the world around you.

To understand Ayurveda and to think Ayurvedically, you need to familiarize yourself with the way the energies of vata, pitta, and kapha manifest themselves in your everyday life. These manifestations can be described in terms of the way we experience them. This book introduces you to the basic principles of Ayurveda, and helps you identify the characteristics, or qualities, of the doshas through a variety of common adjectives you already know, e.g. hot or cold, light or heavy, wet or dry.

This book shows you how to assess the balance of the three doshas in your constitution, and how to decide which dosha predominates. In other words, you can discover whether you are a vata type, a pitta type, or a kapha type. But remember, everything is relative in Ayurveda – these types are starting points for understanding your health.

How is your Constitution Determined?

The state of your parents' doshas at the time you were conceived is primarily responsible for your constitution. This is because the qualities your parents experience in life continuously affect the doshas in every cell of their bodies, including the sperm or ovum.

Let us look at a simple example. Imagine a father-to-be who has a pitta constitution and a pressurized, intellectual job in which he is very ambitious. His current doshic state has even higher pitta than his constitutional balance. The mother-to-be has a kapha constitution and works part time in an undemanding job. She is often bored in the evening waiting for her partner to come home, so she spends her time nibbling and dozing in front of the television. Her kapha energy will be in excess.

All three doshas will be in the baby's constitution, but one, or maybe two, will predominate. If, at the time of conception, the pitta in the father's sperm is stronger than the kapha in the mother's ovum, the baby will have a pitta constitution, with kapha secondary. If the kapha from the ovum dominates, the baby will be kapha, with pitta secondary. If kapha and pitta are of equal strength, the baby will have a pitta–kapha constitution.

Meaning of Ayurveda

Ayurveda is a Sanskrit word which literally means "science of life". "Ayur" means life and "Veda" means science, or knowledge.

In the same way, the state of your doshas and those of your partner will determine the constitution of your offspring. If you and your partner wish to conceive a child, your aim should be to give the baby a well balanced constitution. Factors during pregnancy, such as the mother's diet as well as her physical and emotional health, and the circumstances surrounding the birth experience, can have a secondary influence on the baby's constitution.

The Three Ages of Life

During the cycle of birth to death, we evolve through three different ages, each related to the functions of the doshic energy that predominates in that age. Childhood is the kapha age. The body grows and has a constant demand for nourishment to develop strong tissues. Ailments related to disturbances of kapha are more common in childhood.

The pitta age begins at puberty and lasts through the middle years. Many problems, such as acne, experienced by teenagers can be related to pitta, as this dosha increases in the body. During the pitta age, the body needs to be maintained in a stable state, and conditions due to excess pitta, such as acid indigestion, are more likely. The vata age begins at about 55 years or with the menopause in women. Metabolism begins to slow down and the tissues are not replenished so readily. Often, a dryness in the body precedes more obvious degeneration of the tissues. The correct diet and a regular oil massage can help keep the body supple.

Making Changes

Every day, the ratio of the three doshas within us is altered by whatever we do – eat heavy food, fly on a plane, sit in front of the television for hours, drink lots of coffee in the morning, or stay up all night. So long as the disturbances to our everyday equilibrium are small and not habitual, and so long as we take steps to restore the balance of our constitution, we should remain in health. Once you have a good idea of the doshic nature of your constitution, you

Age and the Doshas

Although one (or perhaps two) of the doshas predominate in your constitution, you will experience a relative increase: in kapha, during your childhood; in pitta, during your middle years; and in vata after the menopause and during old age.

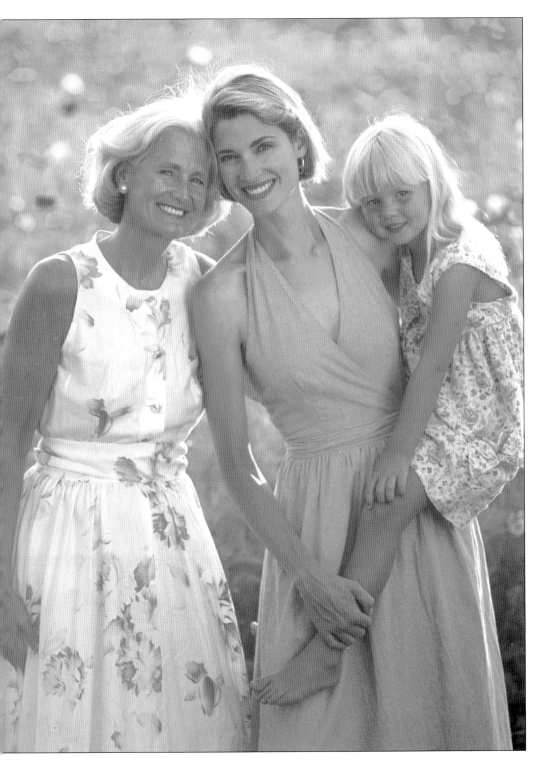

can then go on to establish whether or not your lifestyle is helping you stay healthy.

If the relationship between your vata, pitta, and kapha is disturbed then you will need to take steps to redress the balance and restore the integrity of your constitution. The book contains many charts, lists, and a handful of case studies, or Ayurvedic profiles, to help you establish the details of your lifestyle and to guide you on the changes you may need to make.

In Ayurveda, ill health is related to disturbances of vata, pitta, and kapha in the body. To a trained practitioner, the qualities of the signs and symptoms in the body indicate which dosha is disturbed. For example, excessive dryness in the body is frequently associated with a disturbance of vata, excessive hotness with a disturbance of pitta, and excessive heaviness with a disturbance of kapha. Whatever the signs and symptoms, you will need to adjust your lifestyle and modify some of your habits in order to restore your wellbeing and health.

But how do you adjust your lifestyle? First, you have to discover which dosha is disturbed, and decide what in your lifestyle and diet is causing the disturbance. Then, with your knowledge of qualities uppermost in your mind, select the steps you need to take to restore balance to your doshas. Two crucial principles to remember when planning these changes are: "like increases like" and "opposite qualities decrease". Thus, if your vata dosha is increased and needs to be pacified, do not do things or eat foods that increase vata; instead, select those things and eat those foods that are antagonistic to vata.

Balance and moderation are part of life and health. For example, habitually eating hot spicy food causes the heat in your body and mind to increase. Depending on your constitution and other circumstances in your life, if this heat becomes excessive it could contribute to the disease process – the first signs may have "hot" qualities, such as an

Good Medicine

According to Ayurveda, everything can be a medicine or a poison, depending on how it is used. Moreover, Ayurveda acknowledges that no treatment or remedy is appropriate for all people or in all circumstances. The art of good medicine is two-fold: to understand the patient and their situation; and to know how and when to act to assist nature in bringing appropriate healing to the patient.

itchy rash or an unhelpful, critical attitude of mind. But if you have a "cold" constitution, hot spicy food may help maintain your balance.

As you begin to think Ayurvedically you will understand your uniqueness, your individual requirements in daily life for good health, and how your needs change according to your age, the seasons, and your living circumstances. By understanding the basic principles of Ayurveda you will know how and when to act and what to eat to maintain your health and vitality, and enjoy life up to your constitutional capacity.

Caution:
The guidelines and information provided in this book are not intended to be a substitute for qualified medical advice.

Hot, Spicy Foods
By understanding your current doshic balance, you will know if hot, spicy foods can beneficially be included in your diet.

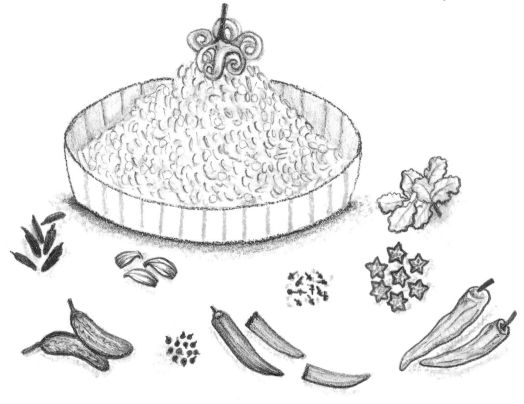

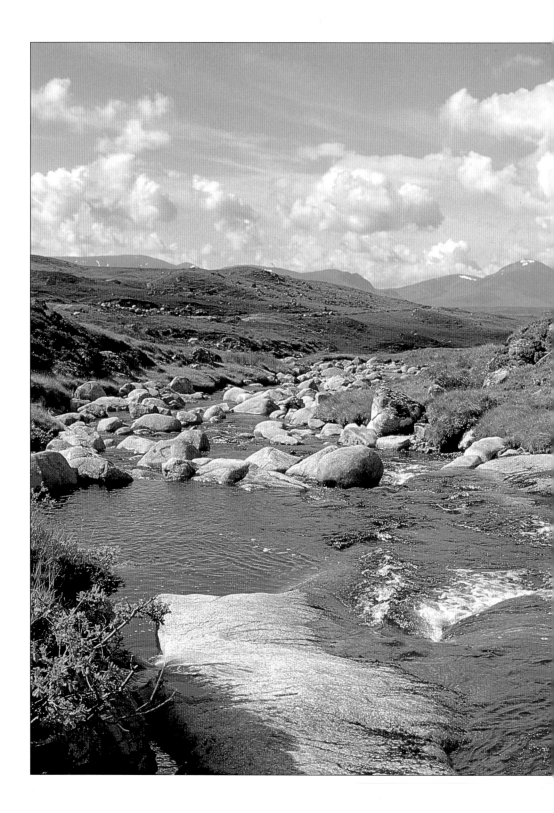

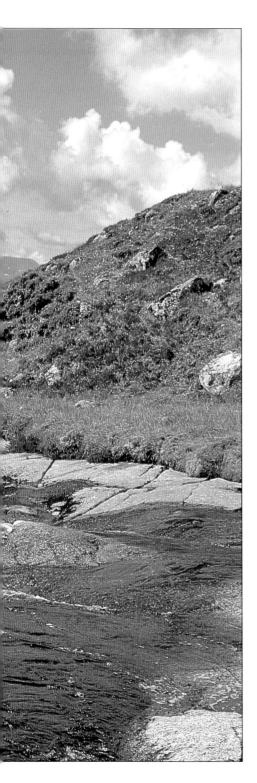

PART ONE

Understanding Ayurveda

The Origins of Ayurveda

व्याधयो हि समुत्पन्नाः सर्वप्राणिभयङ्कराः ।
तद्ब्रूहि मे शमोपायं यथावदमरप्रभो ॥
तस्मै प्रोवाच भगवानायुर्वेदं शतक्रतुः ।
पदैरल्पैर्मतिं बुद्ध्वा विपुलां परमर्षये ॥

*"Diseases causing fear in all living things have appeared, so, O Lord
of god, tell me the proper measures for (their) amelioration."
Then Lord Indra, having observed the wide intelligence of the
great sage, delivered to him Ayurveda in a few words.*
(**Charaka Samhita** *Chapter 1: 18*)

Ayurveda is a traditional healing system of India, with
origins firmly rooted in the culture of the Indian sub-
continent. Some 5000 or more years ago, the great *rishis*, or
seers of ancient India, observed the fundamentals of life
and organized them into a system. Ayurveda was their gift
to us, an oral tradition passed down from generation to
generation.

A few treatises on Ayurveda date from around 1000 BC.
The best-known is *Charaka Samhita*, which concentrates on
internal medicine. Many of today's Ayurvedic physicians
use *Astanga Hrdayam*, a more concise compilation written
over 1000 years ago from the earlier texts. Later texts
include modifications derived from the medical systems of
invading cultures.

Ayurvedic teachings were recorded as *sutras*, succinct
poetical verses in Sanskrit, containing the essence of a
topic and acting as aides-memoire for the students. The
students memorized entire texts, which their *guru*, or
teacher, then brought alive by expounding on the deeper

knowledge contained within the verses. Parts of these texts are available in translation from Sanskrit, but without a teacher they are not readily accessible to Western minds.

Sanskrit, the ancient language of India, reflects the philosophy behind Ayurveda and the depth within it. Sanskrit has a wealth of words for aspects within and beyond consciousness. We lose some of the depths of meaning when we translate the Sanskrit words into Western languages, which cannot deal effectively with all Ayurveda's concepts. Only when concepts, ideas, and inventions enter a culture are words and language developed for them.

पृथिव्यादीनि तत्त्वानि पुरुषान्तानि पञ्चसु ।
क्रमात् कादिषु वर्गेषु मकारान्तेषु सुव्रते ॥
वाय्वग्निसलिलेन्द्राणां धारणानां चतुष्टयम् ।
तदूर्ध्वं शादि विख्यातं पुरस्ताद् ब्रह्मपञ्चकम् ॥
अमूला तत्क्रमाज्ज्ञेया क्षान्ता सृष्टिरुदाहता ।
सर्वेषामेव मन्त्राणां विद्यानां च यशस्विनि ॥
इयं योनिः समाख्याता सर्वतन्त्रेषु सर्वदा ।

The Sanskrit Language
Sanskrit is a beautiful, powerful, resonating language, with a structure and richness not found within most modern languages. The logic and beauty within Sanskrit reflect the two levels needed to appreciate Ayurveda fully: the outer knowledge passed on from teachers and books, and the inner knowledge or intuition gained through experience, by applying what we learn to our daily lives.

THE PHILOSOPHY OF MANIFESTATION

No philosophy has had greater influence on Ayurveda than
Sankhya's philosophy of creation, or manifestation. To use
Ayurveda in your life, you do not have to accept, or even
understand, this philosophy. But if you keep an open mind
toward it, you will gain a deeper insight into the ways
Ayurveda can benefit your health.

According to Sankhya, behind creation there is a state
of pure existence or awareness, which is beyond time and
space, has no beginning or end, and no qualities. Within
pure existence there arises a desire to experience itself,
which results in disequilibrium and causes the
manifestation of primordial physical energy.

This energy is the creative force of action, a source of
form that has qualities. Matter and energy are closely

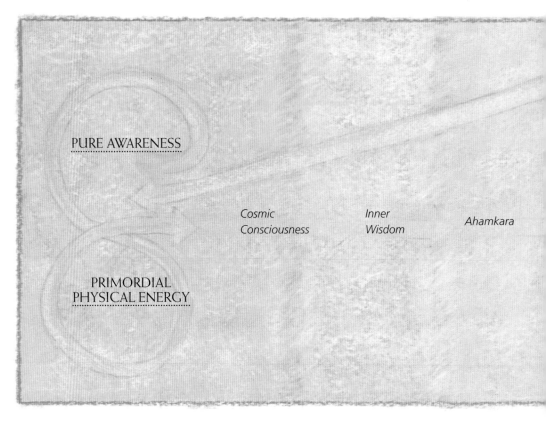

PURE AWARENESS

Cosmic
Consciousness

Inner
Wisdom

Ahamkara

PRIMORDIAL
PHYSICAL ENERGY

related: when energy takes form, we tend to think of it in terms of matter rather than energy. The primordial physical energy is imponderable and cannot be described in words. The most subtle of all energies, it is modified until ultimately our familiar mental and physical world manifests itself.

Pure existence and primordial energy unite for the dance of creation to happen. Pure existence is simply "observing" this dance. Primordial energy and all that flows from it cannot exist except in pure existence or awareness. These concepts of awareness are central to Ayurveda's philosophy and, ultimately, to maintaining health in human beings.

The Energy of Creation
The energy of the dance of creation arises out of pure awareness or existence, the unlimited energy of the universe; this energy is love.

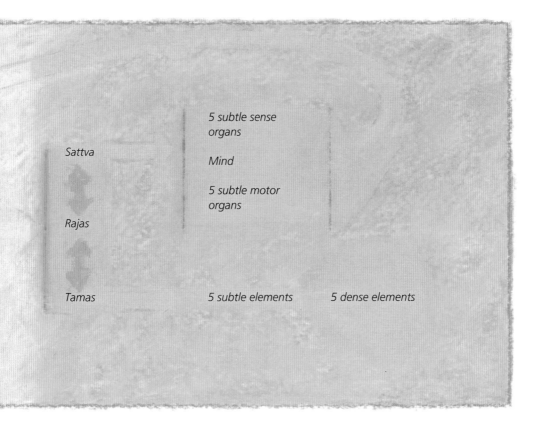

Sattva

Rajas

Tamas

5 subtle sense organs

Mind

5 subtle motor organs

5 subtle elements

5 dense elements

Inner Wisdom

Primordial energy gives rise to cosmic consciousness or intelligence, which is the universal order that pervades all life. Your individual intelligence, which is different from your everyday intellectual mind, is derived from and is part of this cosmic consciousness. It is your inner wisdom: the part of your individuality that cannot be swayed by the demands of daily life or by *ahamkara*, your sense of "I-ness".

Ahamkara is a Sanskrit word with no easy translation; it is a concept that is not fully formed in the West. Sometimes, the word "ego" is equated to ahamkara, but this is misleading, since ahamkara embraces much more. In essence, it is that part of "me" that knows which parts of universal creation are "me". It is my unique vibration to which all physical parts of "me" resonate. "I" am not separate from any part of creation, but "I" have an identity that differentiates and defines the boundaries of "me". All parts of creation have ahamkara, not only human beings.

Elements and Organs

There are five sense organs and five motor organs in the physical body, each have a counterpart in the subtle body. Each of these 10 organs and the five modes of stimuli which correspond to the subtle elements have an affinity to one of the five dense elements (see p. 22).

CONNECTING ELEMENTS WITH ORGANS

Dense Element	Subtle Element	Sense Organ	Motor Organ	Function
Ether	Sound	Ears	Vocal chords	Speaking
Air	Touch	Skin	Hands	Grasping
Fire	Sight	Eyes	Feet	Moving
Water	Taste	Tongue	Genitals	Procreating
Earth	Smell	Nose	Anus	Excreting

Subjective and Objective Worlds

The next part of the philosophy of creation is often difficult for the Western mind to accept, for the concepts are outside what is familiar to most of us, and there is no easy logic to follow.

There arises from ahamkara a two-fold creation: *sattva*, comprising the subjective world, which is able to perceive and manipulate matter; and *tamas*, the objective world of the five elements. *Rajas*, which is the force or energy of movement, brings together parts of both the subjective and objective worlds.

The subjective world comprises the subtle body, which is the mind and the potential for the five sense organs to hear, feel, see, taste, and smell, and for the five organs of action to speak, grasp, move, procreate, and excrete. Your mind and subtle organs are the bridge between your body and your ahamkara and inner wisdom.

This subtle body, together with ahamkara and inner wisdom, is considered the essential nature of humans. Sankhya's philosophy says that there are eight dispositions or fundamental strivings within humans, which are also part of the innermost nature. These are virtue, vice, knowledge, ignorance, non-attachment, attachment, power, and impotence. Until the ultimate knowledge is obtained these strivings are the reason for ordinary existence and suffering. It is this essential, or innermost, nature that "occupies" the physical body.

On a subtle level, the objective world of tamas is sound, touch, vision, taste, and smell – the five subtle elements. These elements give rise to the dense elements – ether, air, fire, water, and earth – from which all matter of the physical world is derived. Even at the stage of the dense elements, the philosophy of creation is still dealing with aspects of existence that are beyond our physical realms. The essential point of this philosophy is that we are first and foremost spirit experiencing existence.

Creation is Now

Sankhya's philosophy of creation is described in stages to aid understanding. In reality, creation, or manifestation, is now and in the present, without past or future. This concept is difficult to comprehend with our everyday mind.

THE GREAT ELEMENTS

In Ayurveda, everything is composed of the five dense elements (often known as the *great* elements) – ether, air, fire, water, and earth. They represent five states, or qualities, of energy or matter. Western science cannot see or measure them, but we know them through the qualities of the energy and matter we experience daily in our physical, mental, and emotional lives.

The elements are everywhere and always together in all things, in an infinite variety of proportions. Although each element has a range of attributes, only some are evident in any particular situation. This variety of proportions and attributes allows for the enormous diversity of life. The five elements are part of the dynamic dance of creation: they are constantly changing and interacting. A change in one element affects the others.

The Elements in Life

All the elements are present in the cell membrane, but the earth element predominates, giving structure to the cell. The water element predominates in the cytoplasm, the liquid in the cell. The metabolic processes regulating the cell are governed mainly by the fire element. The air element predominates in the gases in the cell. The space occupied by the cell represents the ether element.

AIR

The air element is gaseousness, and has airy qualities. It is light, clear, dry, and dispersing.

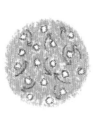

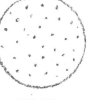

ETHER

Ether is so subtle that we rarely think about it. It is equated to size or space.

FIRE

Fire is the power of change and transformation. It has the qualities of heat, dryness, and upward movement.

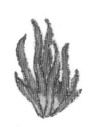

WATER

Water is liquid, cool, and flows downward. It has no shape of its own.

EARTH

Earth is substantial, with the qualities of heaviness, hardness, and only a little downward movement.

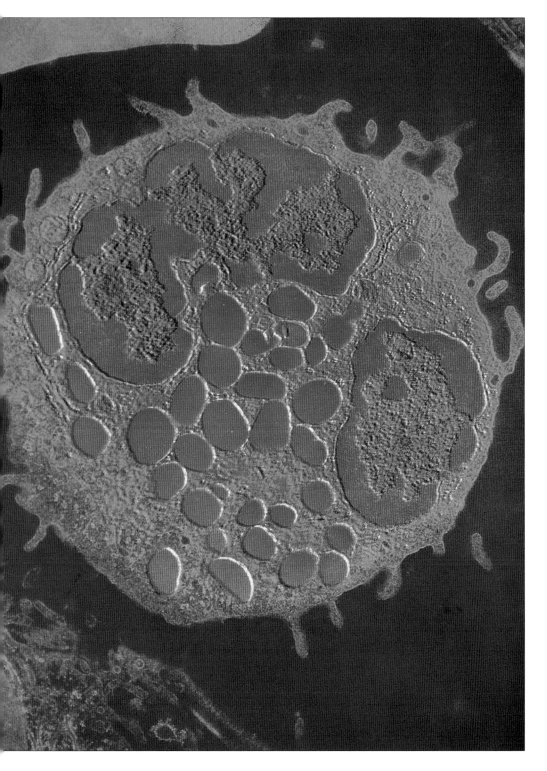

The Fundamental Qualities

Ayurveda is a science of qualities. Although we naturally experience them daily, few in the West are trained to think in terms of qualities and to use our qualitative experiences in an analytical way. To use Ayurveda you need to be able to read qualities in yourself, and in the world around you.

In Ayurveda, subtle and insignificant matters have an influence on a situation. Its philosophy starts at the most subtle level with awareness and then consciousness, which is progressively projected until we can perceive it, with our senses, in its manifested form. These subtle and dense levels interrelate and affect each other through the mind.

Qualitative and quantitative methods of description and analysis do not compete with each other – they are just different models for reality. The secret is to know when, and for what, each is appropriate. Many illnesses are most easily described in terms of experiences and feelings. Fatigue, for example, is hard to define clearly, but may be described with reference to the qualities experienced. In Ayurveda, qualitative descriptions determine what beneficial measures can be taken to restore health.

According to *Charaka Samhita*, we experience everything through 10 pairs of fundamental qualities. Each pair represents the extremes of a continuum (see p. 25). The relationship between a pair of qualities is the basis of two of Ayurveda's fundamental rules. First, that like increases like; second, that a quality is decreased by its opposite quality.

No absolutes exist in the qualitative model, only relativity. Hot is only hot relative to something cooler. To make a qualitative assessment of anything, always take the context and previous circumstances into account. Relationships or interactions between different qualities are also important. One quality can have a different effect on two substances. For example, heat adds a dry quality to bread, but a liquid quality to butter. As you learn to see people in terms of their qualities, it will become clear why each individual is unique, and reacts to stimuli and events in very different ways.

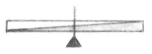

A Pair of Qualities
Each pair of qualities, such as hot and cold, represents the extremes of a continuum. If you take food out of the refrigerator it will be cold. Put it in the freezer and it will become colder – more cold quality has been added. Put it in the oven, adding some hot quality, and the food will become less cold. Leave it in the oven long enough and its temperature will have moved from the cold half of the continuum to the hot half.

The Ten Pairs of Qualities

The traditional text, Charaka Samhita, *lists 20 qualities organized into 10 pairs. Each pair represents two extremes of a continuum and are relative to each other. The two qualities in a pair influence each other.*

Heaviness	Lightness
Coldness	Hotness
Unctuousness	Roughness
Dullness	Sharpness
Stability	Mobility
Softness	Hardness
Non-sliminess	Sliminess
Smoothness	Coarseness
Minuteness	Grossness
Solidity	Liquidity

Elements and Qualities

In Ayurveda, *everything in our world is made up of a combination of the five great elements, which manifest differing aspects and intensities of their qualities. Here, the great elements are related to the fundamental qualities listed by* Charaka Samhita.

QUALITIES OF THE GREAT ELEMENTS

ETHER	AIR	FIRE	WATER	EARTH
Minuteness	Lightness	Hotness	Coldness	Heaviness
	Mobility	Lightness	Liquidity	Solidity
	Roughness	Sharpness	Softness	Stability
		Liquidity	Smoothness	

The Three Vital Energies

वायुः पित्तं कफश्चेति त्रयो दोषाः समासतः ॥
विकृताविकृता देहं घ्नन्ति ते वर्तयन्ति च ।

*Vayu (vata), pitta, and kapha are the three doshas, in brief; they destroy and support
(sustain, maintain) the body when they are abnormal and normal respectively.*
(Astanga Hrdayam *Chapter 1: 6)*

The rishis understood the world in terms of the five great
elements. In creating Ayurveda as a healing system, the
rishis described these elements in a more simplified form as
three vital energies, or doshas. Each dosha is a combination
of two elements. The three doshas are responsible for all
the physiological and psychological processes in your body
and mind. They are dynamic forces that determine growth
and decay. Each of your physical characteristics, mental
capacities, and emotional tendencies can be described in
terms of the three doshas.

The Sanskrit names for the three doshas are vata, pitta,
and kapha. These do not translate easily from Sanskrit.
Your aim should be gradually to learn to recognize the
effects of the doshas in your body and your daily life. The
doshas, like the elements, cannot be detected with our
senses, but their qualities can. They have the qualities of
their two constituent elements, both individually and in
combination. Hence, vata has qualities of air and ether,
plus qualities from a combination of the two.

Vata, pitta, and kapha have specific functions in the body but they do not work in isolation. Full health and wellbeing is only possible when the doshas work harmoniously together. It is important to realize that the three doshas in your being change constantly, due to the doshic qualities of your lifestyle and environment, such as time and season (see pp. 150-1).

When you can recognize the qualities of the doshas in your body and the doshic qualities in your daily life, you will be able to use Ayurveda to maintain them in a healthy balance for you. By learning to distinguish any imbalances, you can use Ayurveda to restore equilibrium to your doshas and so regain full health (see Chapter Four).

The Three Doshas
Each dosha is a combination of two elements, one of which predominates over the other. Often, the three doshas – vata, pitta, and kapha (VPK, for short) – are referred to as the air, fire, and water humours respectively.

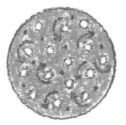

VATA
Vata is a combination of the air and ether elements, with air predominating.

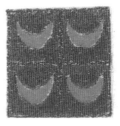

KAPHA
Kapha is a combination of the water and earth elements, with water as the primary element.

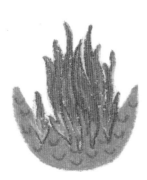

PITTA
Pitta is primarily the fire element, with water as the secondary element.

THE QUALITIES OF VPK

In using Ayurveda it is important to have awareness of the qualities you experience and relate these to the qualities of the doshas. The many nuances in the qualities in your life will be overwhelming, so look initially for broad principles associated with each dosha. For example, the qualities of a windy day sum up vata. The wind is erratic, moves in gusts, dries the washing, and cools you. It is not seen, but its effects are. Heat relates to pitta. A fire gives heat and radiance, and moves upward. Heat melts and penetrates. The two elements of kapha are more equally balanced; the dosha is connected to wet, heavy, or solid qualities. Mud is a useful simile. It is cold and soft, heavy and dense; it might slide slowly downward.

The key words that describe the qualities associated with the doshas are shown on the chart below. Once you have built up a broad picture of qualities for each dosha you can start to think about yourself in doshic terms. You will then be ready to decide what qualities to add or reduce in order to keep your doshas working harmoniously.

Key Words
You will probably grasp the idea of VPK more quickly if you commit this list of key words to memory. Copy the list and display it prominently. Remember that qualities are a continuum – they are always relative rather than absolute, and are experienced in a context, not in isolation.

KEY QUALITIES OF VPK		
VATA (Air and Ether)	PITTA (Fire and Water)	KAPHA (Water and Earth)
Light	Light	Heavy
Cold	Hot	Cold
Dry	Oily	Oily
Rough	Sharp	Slow
Subtle	Liquid	Slimy
Mobile	Sour	Dense
Clear	Pungent	Soft
Dispersing		Static
Erratic		Sweet
Astringent		

When learning about Ayurveda you should first isolate the
concepts of vata, pitta, and kapha to understand their range of
qualities, and only then try to apply the qualities to the complexities of the human mind and body. The qualities of VPK
are listed separately for convenience (see pp. 28, 30-1), but
VPK are not separate energies but different aspects of the
same energy. They are always present together in an infinite
variety of combinations. As your understanding increases you
will appreciate how their qualities overlap and interrelate.

Your body and all your daily experiences are comprised not
of one but many qualities. As you learn to think qualitatively,
look for the main qualities of your feelings and of situations
around you as well as in the physical characteristics of yourself
and those around you. As you gain in confidence and experience in reading qualities, you will eventually become skilled in
distinguishing the subtleties in the qualities you observe.

Qualities of Trees
*The qualities of vata, pitta,
and kapha are all around
us. If you go for a walk
through the woods, see if
you can see these qualities
in different kinds of trees.*

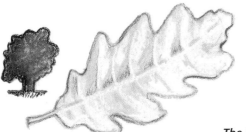

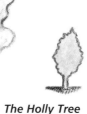

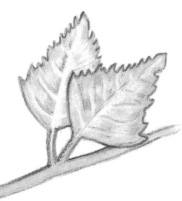

The Oak
*The oak is a kapha tree: large,
sturdy, with a massive trunk,
thick bark, and big branches
that give a full, rounded
silhouette. It is slow growing,
taking perhaps 100 years to
reach maturity.*

The Holly Tree
*The holly tree displays pitta
qualities: smooth, light grey
bark and sharp, spiked leaves.*

The Birch
*The birch has vata qualities: the
tall, thin trunk sways as the
wind blows through its flimsy
branches, and the bark peels
off like dry skin. It grows rapidly to its prime in less than 50
years, but then soon fades.*

QUALITIES OF VPK

This list divides up some of the words we commonly use to describe circumstances in our lives, and assigns them to the key qualities of each dosha.

DISPERSING *dissipating evaporating scattering spreading sprawling*

VATA QUALITIES

ERRATIC *changeable fidgety fitful inconstant irregular kinky spasmodic*

DRY *barren brittle crisp husky non-slimy parched shrivelled wrinkled*

ROUGH *bumpy coarse gritty harsh husky irregular jagged ragged scaly scratchy*

PITTA QUALITIES

SHARP *cutting enquiring inquisitive keen penetrating perceptive piercing pointed quick shrill strong*

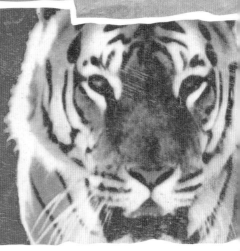

OILY *buttery fat greasy sebaceous slippery smooth unctuous*

KAPHA QUALITIES

COLD *bitter bleak chilled cool freezing glassy icy*

OILY *buttery fat greasy sebaceous slippery smooth unctuous*

HEAVY *chubby dense gross lethargic listless massive obese stodgy*

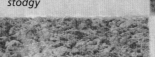

SLOW *dense dull inert lacklustre lingering sleepy slothful tardy torpid*

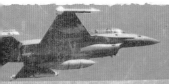

MOBILE *active animated changeable fluid lively moving running swift travelling*

CLEAR *empty obvious transparent*

SUBTLE *discreet hidden imperceptible minute sensitive veiled*

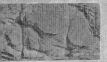

LIGHT *flimsy fluffy fragile skinny thin*

COLD *bitter bleak chilled cool freezing glassy icy*

LIQUID *flowing fluid structureless wet*

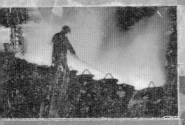

LIGHT *bright fair fire glowing pale radiant*

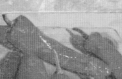

HOT *burning eager fiery inflamed passionate raging scorching sharp spicy sweltering*

SOFT *comfortable creamy cushioning flabby mushy receptive sinking into*

SLIMY *clammy mucusy oily runny slippery smooth soft*

STATIC *calm immobile still*

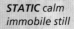

DENSE *dull firm heavy obtuse opaque slow solid thick*

SHARED AND OPPOSING QUALITIES

Each dosha shares a quality with another dosha; the third has the opposite quality. For example, vata and pitta both have a light quality; kapha is heavy. Slight differences exist in the nature of shared qualities. Vata's lightness relates to weight, pitta's to radiance as well as weight. Similarly, both vata and kapha are cold, but vata is dry cold while kapha is wet cold. Vata is not as cold as kapha – for example, a dry, cold climate does not *feel* as cold as a wet, cold climate. Pitta is slightly oily, whereas kapha can be profusely so.

Antagonistic Qualities and Balance

Each dosha has an inherent ability to regulate and balance itself. This ability comes from the antagonistic qualities that arise from the dosha's constituent elements. In vata, for example, one quality of the predominant air element is dispersing but the extent of its dispersal is determined by the space (ether). Too much fire in pitta can evaporate water and have a drying effect; yet too much water quenches fire. In kapha, an increase in the liquid quality makes for a runnier substance, but a relative overabundance of earth element makes a substance more solid.

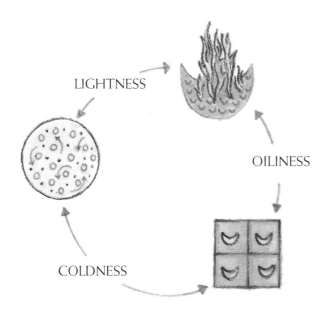

LIGHTNESS

OILINESS

COLDNESS

Shared Qualities

Pitta and kapha share the quality of oiliness and vata has the opposite, dry quality. Vata and kapha share the quality of coldness, whereas pitta is hot. Vata and pitta share the quality of lightness, whereas kapha is heavy. An excess of vata, pitta, or kapha energy in the body is often associated with symptoms that have dry, hot, or heavy qualities respectively.

VPK and your Constitution

Ayurveda is a science of the individual. You are unique, in that only you display the doshas in your way. The ratio of the doshas in your constitution (see p. 9), and the qualities expressed by it, are as unique to every individual as finger-prints. This ratio is the baseline against which you can compare the current levels of your doshas; and it reflects characteristic tendencies and susceptibility to illness.

Although VPK qualities combine in the individual in an infinite number of ways, Ayurveda describes three types of constitution. In mono-types, one dosha predominates: they have either a vata, pitta, or kapha constitution. In duo-types, two doshas have equal strength: they have either vata–pitta, pitta–kapha, or vata–kapha constitutions. In the third type, the three doshas have equal strength. This is rare. When the doshas are well combined, individuals experience excellent health under most circumstances. But if the doshas are poorly combined the individual, however much care he or she takes, suffers illness most of the time.

The uniqueness of an individual arises for two reasons. First, nobody shares exactly the same ratio of vata, pitta, and kapha. Second, no two people manifest the qualities of their doshas in an identical way. You and your friend may both be mono-types, with vata predominating in your con-stitution, but there will be differences in the qualities of the vata and also of pitta and kapha that manifest in you both.

Knowing your constitution (see pp. 38-41) is the first step to anticipating the sort of imbalances that can make you ill and the sort of illnesses you are likely to suffer from. Equally, the knowledge enables you to adjust your life to keep your doshas "balanced", which means maintaining the same ratio of doshas as your constitution. When you have achieved this, you may be able to obtain a better balance which will give you increased vitality. As a rule of thumb, the strongest dosha in your constitution has the greatest tendency to increase, so you will be most susceptible to ill-nesses associated with an increase of that dosha.

CONSTITUTIONAL CHARACTERISTICS

To use Ayurveda to maintain wellness and vitality, you need to know what your constitution is – the original combination of vata, pitta, and kapha in your body. Ideally, you should ascertain this from an expert Ayurvedic physician, who will have been trained in Ayurvedic pulse diagnosis. Your constitution can also be assessed by accurate observation. However, as yet there are few people in the West who have had sufficient training to assess constitution accurately.

Generally, vata characteristics tend to be extreme, irregular, small, light in weight, or dry. Pitta ones will be average or medium, but sharp, quick, and light. Large, heavy, or slow qualities are connected with kapha.

Different Faces
Study the faces around you – family, friends, colleagues, acquaintances. Try to assign their characteristics to V, P, or K, using the descriptions here. Remember, nobody has a face that is completely one dosha or another; everyone is a combination of doshas. Remember, too, that in assessing constitutions all characteristics are taken into account (see pp. 38-41).

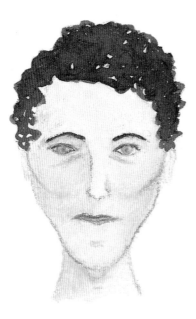

VATA

Vata skin is thin, dry, darkish, and cool, and vata hair is thin, dark, coarse, and either kinky or curly. The face is long and angular, often with an underdeveloped chin. The neck is thin and scrawny. The vata nose is small and narrow, and may be long, crooked, or asymmetrical. Vata eyes are small, narrow, or sunken, dark brown or grey in colour, with a dull lustre. The vata mouth is small, with thin, narrow, or tight lips. Teeth are irregular, protruding, or broken, set in receding gums.

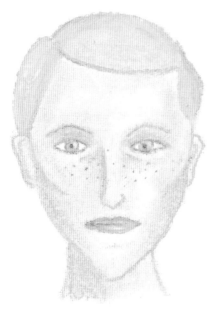

PITTA

Pitta skin is fair, soft, lustrous, and warm, and tends to burn easily in the sun. The skin has freckles, many moles, and a tendency to rashes. Pitta hair is fine and soft, either fair or reddish. The face is heart-shaped, often with a pointed chin. The neck is average and in proportion. The nose is neat, pointed, and average in size. Pitta eyes are average in size, either light blue, light grey, or hazel in colour, with an intense lustre. The pitta mouth is medium with average lips. Teeth are medium-sized and yellowish.

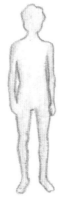

KAPHA

Kapha skin is thick, oily, pale, white, and cold. Kapha hair is plentiful, thick, wavy, lustrous, and generally brown. The face is large, rounded, and full. The neck is solid, with a tree-trunk quality. The kapha nose is large and rounded. Kapha eyes are attractive and large, blue or light brown in colour. The kapha mouth is large with big, full lips. Teeth are big and white, and set in strong gums.

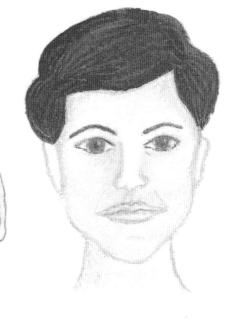

THE DOSHAS AND THE MIND

In Ayurveda, the mind also has a constitution and generally there is a close correlation with your physical constitution. Emotions, too, can be classified into VPK. Individuals have a natural tendency toward certain emotional traits, which will be influenced by their constitution (see also p. 78 and Chapter Seven). As a rule, you will feel positive emotions more readily when your doshas are balanced.

Positive States
This list classifies our positive mental and emotional states according to VPK. Your current doshic balance will affect how you think and feel at present. Use this list in conjunction with the qualities on pp. 30-1.

VATA

Creativity ~ Enthusiasm ~
Freedom ~ Generosity ~
Joy ~ Vitality
If you have a vata constitution, you are likely to be artistic and creative with a good imagination, though you may find it hard to put your ideas into practice, as new ideas continually catch your imagination. Your memory may not be very good.

PITTA

Ambition ~ Concentration ~ Confidence ~
Courage ~ Enthusiasm for knowledge ~
Happiness ~ Intelligence
A pitta constitution generally means you have a very alert, focussed mind. You grasp information quickly and manipulate it to your advantage. Your memory is good for information you consider useful for furthering your aims, but not so good at remembering birthdays and anniversaries.

KAPHA

Caring ~ Centredness ~ Compassion
Contentment ~ Faith ~ Fulfilment
Groundedness ~ Patience ~
Sense of being nourished ~ Stability
Support ~ Tenderness
If kapha predominates in your constitution, you will have a steady and reliable mind. You may take time to learn, but will remember what you have learnt. There can sometimes be an element of dullness with a kapha mind; it is usually content not to seek fresh mental stimulation.

The Gift of Love
Love is unconditional and universal. It cannot be affected by physical, emotional, or mental states, though your ability to receive and give love can be.

Normal Functions of VPK

Vata, pitta, and kapha have specific functions in the body and mind. Vata is mobile, and is involved in all movements, large and small. Pitta is hot; its chief function is the metabolic transformations in the body and assimilation of mental experiences. Kapha is the body's supply system and also provides lubricating fluids such as mucus.

VATA

Stimulation of nerves
Transmission of sensory stimuli
Initiation of motor functions
Creation of impulses
Creation of reflexes
Maintenance of consciousness
   through prana, the life force
Inspiration and expiration
Heart beats
Circulation of blood, oxygen,
   nutrients, thoughts
Stimulation of digestive juices
Peristalsis
Normal elimination
Normal transformation of
   tissues
Ejaculation
Delivery of fetus from womb
Stimulation of tears
Expression of emotion
Enthusiasm
Creativity

PITTA

All transformations within the mind and body
Digestion, absorption, and assimilation of food
Maintenance of body temperature
Creation of hunger and thirst
Lustre of eyes and skin
Vision
Comprehension of sensory stimuli
Assimilation of thoughts
Recognition
Discrimination
Intellect, comprehension, and reasoning
   capacity
Confidence
Cheerfulness

KAPHA

Protection, e.g. mucous lining of stomach
Unctuousness
Lubrication, e.g. synovial fluid in joints
Binding, firmness, heaviness in the body
Softness in the body
Distribution of heat
Strength and stamina

Longevity of cells and thus the person
Sleep
Long-term memory
Groundedness and security
Compassion
Absence of greed

CONSTITUTIONAL ASSESSMENT

The charts on the next three pages are designed to help you assess your constitution. Look at the entries in the left hand column and then assess whether you are vata, pitta, or kapha for that particular characteristic. If the concepts of vata, pitta, and kapha are new to you, repeat the assessment as your understanding of the doshas increases in order to get a more accurate result.

Be honest and observant; judge how you are, not how you would like to be. Look for trends that endure. For example, if your weight has been average for 40 years but has increased recently, the gain is likely to be due to lifestyle rather than constitution. Make the assessments in relation to your ethnic background. Ask a friend who knows you well to check your assessments. Take time to reflect on the questions but not for so long that too many details sway your judgment. Rely on the answer that comes to you after honest consideration.

No one is purely vata, pitta, or kapha. To get an accurate assessment you may need to assess secondary influences. For example, a sharp pointed nose will be pitta, but if it is slightly larger than average then there will be a secondary kapha influence.

Guidelines for Filling in the Charts
- *Photocopy the following pages to fill in the charts.*
- *For each entry place a tick over the doshic description that best describes you as you are or have been for most of your life. If you fall equally between two descriptions, tick both.*
- *If you detect a strong secondary influence mark it with a cross.*
- *Leave any items that you do not know, e.g. fertility.*
- *There are no right or wrong answers. Use the information as a guide to help you understand your unique combination of the doshas.*
- *Take your time to consider the qualities in the assessment. Treat it as a learning exercise. Before you start, look at the questions in relation to people around you. This will help you to see the doshas and enable you to recognize your own qualities. You will also begin to realize that the descriptions are all relative – you may even see yourself in a different way once you notice the qualities in others.*

Assessing the Ticks and Crosses
- *Everyone has vata, pitta, and kapha in their constitution so you should have ticks in all three columns and crosses in some.*
- *When you have finished the assessment, add up the total number of ticks and crosses for each column in each of the four assessments (physical build, physical characteristics, etc). The dosha with the highest number of ticks should be your constitutional type.*
- *If the highest two doshas are very close, look at the number of crosses under each. The one with substantially more crosses than the other might be your constitutional type; or else you have a duo-type of constitution (see p. 33).*
- *If the totals for all three are very close, and no one column has substantially more crosses, then put greater emphasis on your answers under physical build and characteristics as these are the most stable and least affected by lifestyle changes. Repeat the assessment when you are more experienced in reading qualities – an equal ratio of the doshas is rare.*

PHYSICAL BUILD

	V	P	K
Size at birth	Small	Average	Large
Height	Exceptionally short or tall (bean-pole)	Medium	Tall and sturdy, or short and stocky
Weight	Light. Difficulty putting on weight	Moderate. No problem gaining or losing weight	Heavy. Finds it hard to lose weight
Frame/bone structure	Light, delicate. Hips/ shoulders narrow	Medium	Large. Broad shoulders/big hips
Joints	Prominent, dry, knobbly	Normal. Well proportioned	Big. Well formed and lubricated
Musculature	Slight. Prominent tendons	Medium. Firm	Plentiful. Solid
Ticks	*Total*	*Total*	*Total*
Crosses	*Total*	*Total*	*Total*

PHYSICAL CHARACTERISTICS

	V	P	K
Skin	Thin, dry, darkish. Cool	Fair, soft, lustrous, warm. Freckles. Many moles	Thick, oily, pale or white. Cold
Hair	Thin, dark, coarse, kinky or curly	Fine, soft, fair or reddish	Plentiful, thick, wavy, lustrous, generally brown
Shape of face	Long, angular. Chin often under-developed	Heart-shaped. Chin often pointed	Large, rounded, full
Neck	Thin. Very long or very short	Average. In proportion	Solid, tree trunk quality
Nose	May be crooked, small, or narrow	Neat, pointed, average in size	Large, rounded
Eyes – size	Small, narrow, or sunken	Average	Large, prominent
Eyes – colour	Dark brown or grey	Light blue or grey, hazel	Blue or light brown
Eyes – lustre	Dull	Intense	Attractive
Teeth	Irregular, protruding. Receding gums.	Medium size, yellowish	White, big. Strong gums
Mouth	Small Receding gums	Medium	Large
Lips	Thin, narrow, tight	Average	Big, full
Ticks	*Total*	*Total*	*Total*
Crosses	*Total*	*Total*	*Total*

PHYSIOLOGICAL FUNCTIONS

	V	P	K
Sweat	Minimal	Profuse, especially when hot. Strong fleshy or sour smell	Moderate, but present even when not exercising
Temperature preferences	Craves warmth	Loves coolness	Dislikes cold
Sleep	Light, fitful	Sound but short	Deep, likes plenty

PHYSIOLOGICAL FUNCTIONS Continued

	V	P	K
Stools and elimination	Irregular, constipated. Hard, dry stools	Regular. Loose stools	Slow elimination, plentiful and heavy
Activity level	Always doing many things, fidgets	Moderate	Lackadaisical
Endurance	Expends energy quickly, and sinks until recovered	Manages energy well	Good stamina
Sexual arousal	Intense; quickly expended. Fantasizes	Strong; desires and actions matched	Slow; then passion maintained
Fertility	Low	Average	Good
Speech	Fast talking	Sharp, clear, precise	Slow, maybe laboured
Ticks	**Total**	**Total**	**Total**
Crosses	**Total**	**Total**	**Total**

PSYCHOLOGICAL ASPECTS

	V	P	K
Thinking	Superficial with many ideas. More thoughts than deeds	Precise, logical. Good planner and gets plans carried out	Calm, slow, cannot be rushed. Good organizer
Memory	Poor long-term	Good, quick	Good long-term, takes time to learn.
Deep beliefs	Changes these frequently, according to latest mood	Extremely strong convictions that may govern behaviour	Deep steady beliefs that are not easily changed
Emotional tendencies	Fearful, anxious, insecure	Angry, judgmental	Greedy, possessive
Work	Creative	Intellectual	Caring
Lifestyle	Erratic	Busy, but plans to achieve much	Steady and regular. Maybe stuck in a rut
Ticks	**Total**	**Total**	**Total**
Crosses	**Total**	**Total**	**Total**

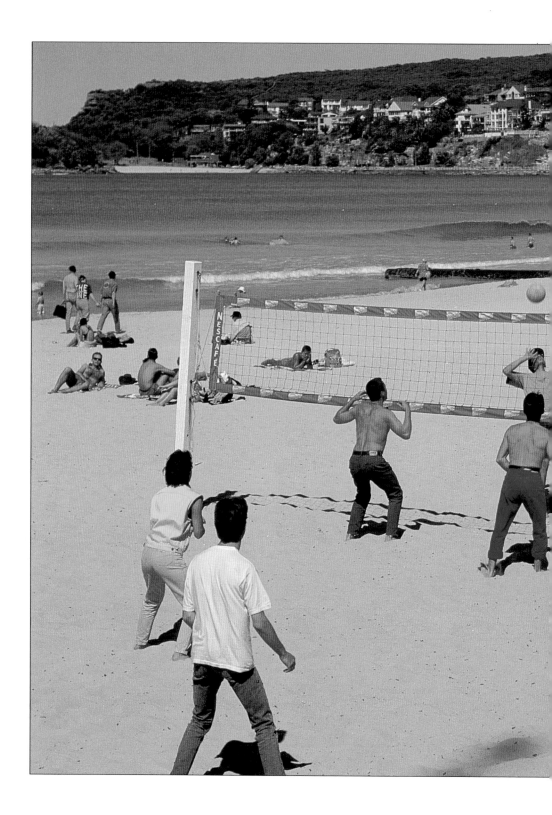

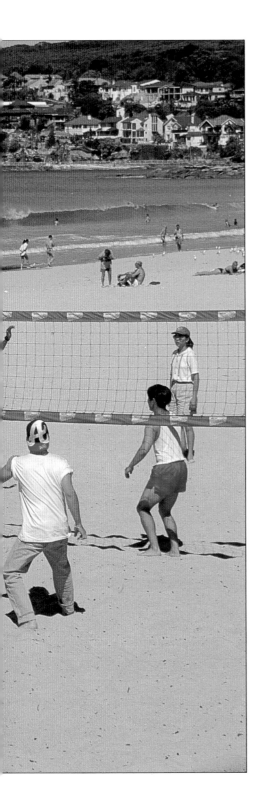

Part Two

The Body in Health and Disease

The Body in Health

दोषधातुमला मूलं सदा देहस्य............ ।

Doshas, dhatus (tissues) and malas (waste products) are the roots (causes, chief constituents, supports) of the body always (throughout the span of life).
(**Astanga Hrdayam** *Chapter 11: 1*)

Ayurveda says we each reflect every aspect of creation. Like a hologram, each part potentially contains the knowledge of the whole, the smaller being reproduced in the image of the greater. The universe is the macrocosm, and nested within are human beings, or microcosms.

According to Sankhya's philosophy (see pp. 18-21), all matter, including our bodies, consists of the five great elements. The physical structure and functions of the body are also understood in terms of the three doshas (see p. 37), as are aspects of our emotional and mental processes.

In health, the doshas work together to produce strong, healthy tissues and good powers of digestion, assimilation, and elimination. When the doshas are in balance the mind and body will be in harmony, producing emotional stability and good mental faculties.

The key to using Ayurveda is knowing how vata, pitta, and kapha work in the body, and how they are affected by influences from both inside and outside the body. These influences include the state of your metabolism, what you eat and do each day, how you think and feel, and the climate and environment in which you live and work. Understanding and recognizing vata, pitta, and kapha's roles in the healthy body will help you understand how they are involved in disease and ill health.

Ayurveda primarily describes the functions and sequences of refinements of tissues in the body. It also describes a subtle system of energy channels, or *nadis*, similar to the meridians in Chinese medicine.

VPK in the Body

You need to consider two main aspects of the doshas when looking at the body in health. First and foremost is the unique balance of the doshas in your body – your constitution (see pp. 38-41). Second is the range of each dosha's normal functions (see p. 37) and the areas of the body with which the doshas have a special affinity (see pp. 46-7).

As you examine the functions of vata, pitta, and kapha in the body, refer back to the list of the doshas' qualities on pages 30-1; this will help you see the way Ayurveda is organized. You may find that a number of paradoxes and ambiguities arise. But if you keep an open, enquiring mind you allow opportunities for insights.

At this stage, do not be tempted to draw conclusions about your health. You will need to let your understanding deepen first, as you learn to think from the Ayurvedic perspective. As with any new skill you need to start with the broad principles and cannot expect to know everything immediately. The skill comes with practice as does judging which factors are most important for you and your body. You are already familiar with your body, and can learn to relate how you feel physically and emotionally to the qualities of the doshas. Reading your body through qualities requires clear observation and experience. You need to understand the qualities in the whole context of your spirit, mind, body, and environment. You should not draw conclusions from one factor alone.

Elements in the Body

Vata (air/ether) is mainly concerned with movement, and the space in which it happens. Pitta (fire/water) is linked to metabolism and its secretions. Kapha (water/earth) gives the body structure and solidity.

Ether	All cavities, e.g. abdominal cavity
Air	Movement, breath
Fire	Enzymes, hormones
Water	Liquid tissues, e.g. lymph
Earth	Solid tissues

Classifying parts of the body into VPK seems to contain ambiguities. Don't dismiss these for they are a reflection of the different levels of understanding in Ayurveda. For example, bones can be related to the earth element as they give structure and support to the body. But on page 47, you will see that they are a subsidiary site of vata. This is because bones are porous and the spaces in them are related to ether, one of the vata elements.

Seats of Vata, Pitta, and Kapha

As different aspects of one energy the doshas are always
together. However, each dosha is associated with particular
parts of the body, places where its force tends to predominate. First and foremost, each dosha has a main place, or
seat, in a part of the gastro-intestinal tract.

   One major role of the seat is to accommodate the small
daily changes in the dosha without significantly disturbing
the body's functioning. The small "excesses" of a dosha (see
pp. 62-3) are held in its seat and expelled from the body
via the gastro-intestinal tract. But accumulation of excessive
dosha in its "seat" is part of the early stage of the disease
process (see pp. 68-9).

Seats of the Doshas
*The seat, or main place, of
each dosha is in the gastro-
intestinal tract.*

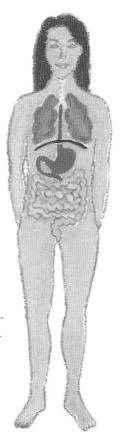

KAPHA
*The stomach and also the
lungs are the seat of kapha.*

VATA
The colon is the seat of vata.

PITTA
*The stomach and the small
intestines are the seat of pitta.*

SUBSIDIARY SITES

In addition to its seat, each dosha has a special affinity with
subsidiary sites (see below), which are closely related to its
functions (see p. 37). For example, a subsidiary site of vata,
which is responsible for the movement of the body, is the
nervous system. The gallbladder and thus bile are linked
with pitta and digestion. One function of kapha is lubrication, which is related to the synovial fluid in joints.

KAPHA

Mucous membranes
Plasma and lymph
Cytoplasm (in cells)
White matter (in brain)
*Joints (synovial membrane
    and fluid)*
Subcutaneous fat
Mouth
Nose
*All secretions,
    e.g. mucus, saliva*

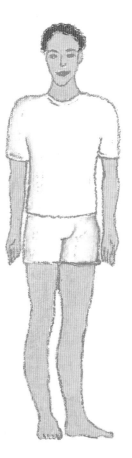

VATA

Pelvic cavity
Lower back
Thighs
Bones
Ears
Skin
Nervous system
Cavities, e.g. ear canal

PITTA

Liver
Spleen
Gall bladder
Blood
Sweat
Eyes
Endocrine glands, e.g. pituitary

AGNI

In Ayurveda, *agni* encompasses changes or refinements in the body and mind from the dense to the more subtle. Such changes include the digestion and absorption of food in the gastro-intestinal tract and cellular transformations, as well as the assimilation of sensory perceptions and mental and emotional experiences. As such, agni covers whole sequences of chemical interactions and changes in the body and mind. Your "digestive" abilities on all levels are related to the strength of your agni.

Agni and pitta are closely connected. Agni and pitta are both hot and light but the other qualities of agni are subtle and dry. According to Dr. Vasant Lad in his book *Ayurveda: The Science of Self-Healing*, "Pitta contains heat energy, which helps digestion. This heat energy is agni". The strength of the body to resist disease and also your physical strength are the outcome of this heat-energy, which determines the metabolic processes of the body.

Balanced agni is vital for health. Ayurveda regards disturbances to agni as one of the chief causes of disease (see pp. 76-7). You must take your power to digest food into account when deciding what is the correct diet for you (see Chapter Six).

Ayurveda describes various agnis in the body and mind according to the conversion or transformation made. The main agni is the gastric fire, responsible for digesting the food we eat and turning it into substances that the body can absorb. This agni correlates with the hydrochloric acid in the stomach and the digestive enzymes and juices secreted into the stomach, duodenum, and small intestines. If your digestive agni is low, your digestive capacity will be impaired: you may experience pain, discomfort or a feeling of heaviness after eating, gases, gurglings, constipation, or loose stools (see pp. 76-7).

THE DIGESTIVE PROCESS

Good digestion is vital for health. To achieve it, you need
to understand your digestion and eat according to your
agni, i.e. digestive capacity. The alternative – indigestion or
incomplete digestion – leads to *ama* (see p. 77) and the disturbance of one or more of the doshas. According to
Ayurveda, this is a root cause of illness.

Often, we only think about our digestive organs when
we experience discomfort. Digestion is your body's means
of "cooking", or transforming, food into a form that can be
absorbed. If you digest your food fully, it will be absorbed
and assimilated by the body and used to build strong,
healthy tissues (see pp. 56-7).

Your digestive ability is related to the strength of your
agni. Poor digestion leads to malabsorption and the
absorption of undigested or incompatible products that
result in ama, clogged channels, inferior tissues, and
disturbed doshas. One indication of malabsorption is teeth
indentations on the sides of the tongue.

Digestion within the body starts in the mouth. Food
stimulates your taste buds and your smell receptors. These
perceptions, via the brain, influence how much and which
digestive juices (agni) are secreted in the stomach and small
intestines. The breakdown of the food begins with chew-
ing, which mixes it with saliva. The more juice-like each
mouthful is when swallowed the better: the particles are
smaller, thereby increasing the food's surface area, which
allows the digestive fluids to act upon them more effectively. This first stage of digestion is related to kapha and food
that is well masticated is associated with the sweet taste
(see pp. 52-5).

Your stomach mixes food with digestive enzymes and
hydrochloric acid, which is capable of burning – the "fire"
of digestion. This is the beginning of the pitta activity of
transforming what was external into an integral part of you.
The length of time food remains in the stomach depends
on the individual and the nature and amount of food eaten.

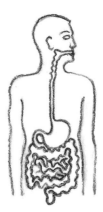

Pain during Digestion
*The stages of the digestive
process are related to vata,
pitta, and kapha. If you
experience discomfort or
pain during digestion, note
how long after eating the
pain arrives. Pain soon after
eating, whilst food is in the
stomach, indicates imbal-
anced kapha. Pain two to
four hours after eating may
involve a pitta problem.
Flatulence or discomfort
some time after eating is a
sign of disturbed vata.
Remember not to read
single signs or symptoms in
isolation.*

For example, melons pass through the stomach more quickly than cereals. Consequently, if you eat melons at the same meals as cereals, the cereals may not be properly digested. In the intestines, bile and other digestive enzymes continue the process, transforming the food and preparing it for absorption. If absorption is impaired you do not obtain all the nutrients, nor any supplements, from your food. However, a simple, easily digestible diet facilitates absorption. The digestion in the stomach and small intestines is associated with pitta and the sour and salt tastes (see pp. 52-5). This corresponds with the release of enzymes and bile salts. At a later stage of digestion, in the ileum, the predominant taste is pungent.

The colon continues the absorption process, particularly of water, calcium, and other minerals. According to Ayurveda, the colon absorbs prana, the life force, which we obtain from breath and food. Prana from food supplies the body's long-term reservoir of this vital life force. If you habitually eat foods with insufficient prana – for example, food that is stale or over-processed – or if your colon's ability to absorb prana is impaired (e.g. by flatulence or clogged channels), then your vitality may be low and this may lead to fatigue. The final stages of digestion are associated with vata and the bitter and astringent tastes.

Regular and complete elimination of feces (see pp. 126-7) is the last part of the digestive process, preparing the system for further supplies of nutrients.

Agni

The literal translation of agni is fire, and fire transforms completely that which it consumes.

Digestive Requirements

Fruit should not be eaten with foods that have different digestive requirements. For example, you should avoid eating melons with other foods because the fruit passes through the stomach more quickly.

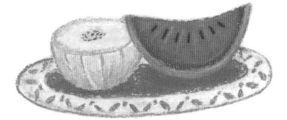

THE THREE STAGES OF DIGESTION

Ayurveda describes the digestion of food in three stages related to the effects on the body. These are "tastes", or the immediate effect; "energetics", or medium-term effect; and the "post-digestive", or long-term, effect.

In Ayurveda, "taste" has an extended meaning and does not just refer to the perceptions on the tongue. Ayurveda says there are six tastes: sweet, sour, salty, pungent, bitter, and astringent (see pp. 54-5). The six tastes also include the effects substances and experiences have within the body and are also related to the five great elements (see chart below). When first encountered, you may find this way of looking at food and digestion difficult to comprehend. As your understanding of Ayurveda deepens you will see the relationship between the subtle aspects, through the elements, doshas, and tastes, of digestion and food to your physical, mental, and emotional wellbeing.

The immediate effect of putting food or drink in your mouth is the sensory stimulation of taste on your tongue. The perception of taste is within the eater, not the food. Your perception of taste will be affected by what you

Tastes and Elements
There are six tastes (see pp. 54-5), each a combination of two elements. Tastes either increase or reduce the doshas, digestion, and the body tissues. For example, the sweet taste (earth/water) increases kapha, slows digestion, and increases weight.

CONNECTING TASTES WITH ELEMENTS

Taste	Great elements	Vata	Kapha	Pitta	Energetics	PDE
Sweet	Earth & water	P	I	P	C	Sweet
Sour	Fire & earth	P	I	I	H	Sour
Salty	Water & fire	P	I	I	H	Sweet
Pungent	Fire & air	I	P	I	H	Pungent
Bitter	Air & ether	I	P	P	C	Pungent
Astringent	Air & earth	I	P	P	C	Pungent

P = pacifies   I = increases   C = cooling   H = heating

habitually eat, your doshic preferences, the tastes your body needs, and what you have recently consumed. Coffee, for example, is bitter and makes other foods more palatable. It is sometimes drunk with very sweet foods to reduce their sweetness.

The "energetics" of food influence the digestive process, either enhancing it or slowing it (and also the body) down. Energetics are either heating or cooling. Foods with heating energetics are more easily digested, generally increasing pitta and pacifying kapha and vata. Foods with cooling energetics give rise to slower, heavier digestion and they tend to decrease pitta and increase kapha and vata.

The general rule is that sour, salty, and pungent foods are heating and, except in excess, will aid digestion. Sweet, bitter, and astringent tastes are cooling and slow down digestion. There are exceptions – for example, honey is sweet but heating.

"Post-digestive" effects (PDE) are the long-term effects that substances have on the body. They can be either anabolic (increasing tissues and thus weight) or catabolic (breaking down or depleting tissues). There are three categories of PDE – sweet, sour, and pungent (these refer to the effects on the body (see pp. 54-5), not the taste on the tongue). Foods with sweet and salty tastes have sweet PDE, which increases tissues. Sour-tasting foods are sour in PDE, while pungent, bitter, and astringent tastes have pungent PDE. Sour and pungent PDE reduce or dry up body tissue.

Special Actions

Some substances, mainly herbs and substances used in Ayurvedic medicine, do not comply with the rules about tastes, energetics, and PDE; they have their own special actions, or prabhav in Sanskrit, which are known through long usage. The versatility of Ayurvedic herbology comes from the detailed knowledge of these rules and prabhav of substances.

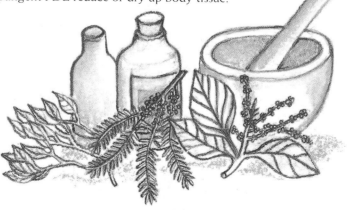

ACTIONS OF THE SIX TASTES

The Sanskrit text, Astanga Hrdayam, *describes the characteristics of the six tastes and the problems that might be experienced from habitual over-consumption of foods of a particular taste. Most foods are a combination of two or more of these tastes, e.g. coffee is bitter and pungent.*

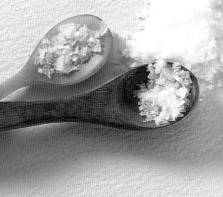

SWEET TASTE

Mitigates P and V • Produces greater strength in the tissues • Valuable for the aged, wounded, emaciated, and children • Universally liked, often adheres to the inside of the mouth, and gives feelings of pleasure, contentment, and comfort • Good for complexion, hair, senses, ojas • Increases breast milk • Unites broken parts such as bones • Prolongs life and helps life activities • Excess use may produce diseases arising from fat and excess kapha, e.g. obesity, dyspepsia, unconsciousness, diabetes, enlargement of neck glands, or malignant tumours

SOUR TASTE

Increases P and K • Stimulates agni • Good for heart and digestion • Encourages inactive vata energy in the pelvic cavity to move downward, aiding elimination • Sets teeth on edge, increases salivation • Excess use may cause looseness or flabbiness, loss of strength, giddiness, itching, irritation, a whitish yellow pallor, herpetiform lesions, swellings, thirst, fever, and diseases arising from excess pitta or kapha

SALT TASTE

Increases P and K • Clears obstructions of the channels and pores • Increases digestive activity and salivation • Lubricates and causes sweating • Penetrates the tissues • Improves taste • Excess use may cause baldness, greying of the hair, wrinkles, thirst, skin diseases, blood disorders, herpetiform lesions, loss of body strength

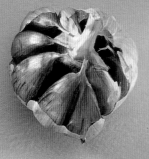

PUNGENT TASTE

Increases V and P, mitigates K • Increases hunger, is digestive, and improves taste • Causes irritation, brings secretions from the eyes, nose, mouth, and gives burning feeling in the mouth • Pungent foods include onion, garlic, and chillies • Dries up the moisture of food • Breaks up hard masses, dilates the channels • Excess use may cause thirst, depletion of reproductive tissue and strength, fainting, contracture, tremors, pain in the waist and back, and other disorders due to excess vata or pitta

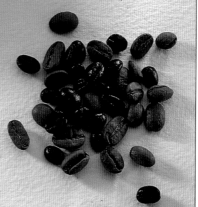

BITTER TASTE

Mitigates P and K • Not liked by itself • Dries up moisture from fat, muscles, feces, urine • Cleans the mouth, destroys taste perception • Bitter herbs and spices include fenugreek seeds • Said to cure anorexia, worms, bacteria, parasites, thirst, skin diseases, loss of consciousness, fever, nausea, burning sensations • Excess use increases vata, causing diseases of vata origin and depletion of the tissues

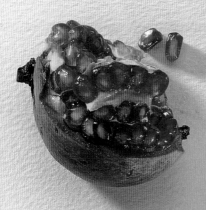

ASTRINGENT TASTE

Increases V • Mitigates increased P and K • Cleans the blood • Causes healing of ulcers • Dries up moisture and fat • Absorbs water, causing constipation and dryness • Hinders digestion of undigested food • Diminishes taste perception and causes a choking sensation • Astringent foods include unripe bananas, pomegranates, chick peas • Excess use causes stasis of food without digestion, flatulence, pain in the cardiac region, emaciation, loss of virility, obstruction of channels, and constipation

THE SEVEN TISSUES

The tissues are the body's structure. Ayurveda classifies them by the way they are produced, as a series of transformations and refinements within the body. There are seven tissue types, with primary and secondary "by-products". Broadly, the types are: plasma and lymph; blood; muscle; fat; bone; bone marrow and nerve tissue; and reproductive tissue. These terms are not entirely accurate, since they do not correspond exactly to the original Sanskrit. The blood tissue, for instance, includes blood vessels and all tissues connected with the blood system.

The by-products are tissues or substances that are either used in the body, or expelled by it once they have served their purpose. In assessing the health of each tissue type the amount and quality of the by-products are taken into account, since they give information about the tissues and the doshas. Scanty menses, for example, will indicate to an Ayurvedic practitioner that the first tissue type (plasma and lymph) may be affected by excess vata. Each tissue type has its own agni (see p. 48), which equates to the enzymes and other secretions needed to create the tissue.

The Tissue Transformation Sequence

An analogy to explain the manner in which the tissues are produced is a series of seven related factories (see right), each generating one of the tissue types and the "raw materials" for the next factory.

Under this arrangement, the product of the seventh factory is the most refined, as its raw materials have already undergone a number of processes. Many days go by after the first factory receives its raw materials before the seventh factory can complete its product. Each factory is dependent on the previous ones. If the processing is not right in one factory the amount or the quality of its products will be affected, which will affect the functioning of the other factories further down the line. Later factories will be affected if earlier ones produce insufficient raw

OJAS

Ancient texts say there are eight drops of ojas in the heart. A subtle substance on the border between mind and body, it maintains life and is closely related to immunity. The West has no concept of ojas; it literally means vitality or bodily strength. Illness arises from the low production or depletion of ojas. According to Charaka Samhita, causes of diminution of ojas include excessive exercise, fasting, loss of blood and semen, anxiety, fear, grief, and injuries. Excessive sexual activity reduces ojas in both sexes. Diminished ojas reduces the body's immunity. It also makes you fearful, emaciated, causes disorders of the sense organs, and impairs mental abilities.

naturally accommodate small changes in the doshas through their seats (see p. 46).

Problems begin when your body's ability to cope with excess qualities has been over-extended, or when your mind does not accept experiences, or when you need more time to adjust to changes. At this point, you should take active steps to restore the natural harmony of your being.

Ayurveda's concept of the disease process is logical. The doshas are energy. The right amount of the right kind of energy at the right time produces the right results. Too much or too little energy, or the wrong type, or at the wrong time, or in the wrong place, and your system will suffer adversely.

Generally, a diet and lifestyle inappropriate to your con-stitution will cause your doshic levels to increase slowly. However, if you suffer traumas, such as bereavement, acci-dents, sudden life changes, surgery, or become a victim of crime, these levels can change dramatically. The effect of such doshic changes depends on the state of your doshas, mind, and body.

Your doshic balance can be disturbed by depleted agni and by the production and/or accumulation of toxins in the body. By understanding the qualities of various signs in the mind and body you will learn about any doshic imbalances that you are experiencing. But first you need to understand your constitutional balance (see pp. 38-41) – this is your baseline against which you can assess any imbalance.

VPK and the Seasons
Each dosha is naturally increased during the season that has similar qualities (see also p. 150). You should take extra care to keep your predominant dosha pacified during its season. In addition, your doshas may be more easily disturbed at the junctions between seasons.

Doshic Imbalance

You have a unique balance of doshas – your constitution –
which is determined at conception. When the current ratio
of your doshas is different from your constitution your
doshas are out of balance. Words used in the West to
describe out of balance doshas include high, low, increased,
decreased, excessive, disturbed, deranged, provoked, aggravated. The changes in doshic states are relative, and all the
circumstances must be considered. Hot, spicy foods
increase pitta and decrease vata and kapha, but it is when
you have eaten an excessive amount for *you* that your pitta
dosha is aggravated. The same food may help pacify your
kapha dosha if it is excessive, or perhaps maintain your balance if you have a vata constitution.

All your experiences have qualities, each related to the
qualities of vata, pitta, and/or kapha. A dosha is increased
by those experiences that have similar qualities to the
doshas and decreased by opposing qualities. Something
with opposing qualities may "pacify" an increased dosha.
So, how does one of your doshas become imbalanced? The
answer is when you experience too many of a particular
dosha's qualities without enough of their opposite qualities
(see p. 32) to pacify or reduce the excessive doshic energy.

A key to understanding Ayurveda is to realize that you
are most susceptible to increases in the dosha that predominates in your constitution. Remember, like attracts like. For
example, if you have a pitta constitution, pitta qualities predominate in you. You will have a natural inclination toward
those things that also have pitta qualities, thus increasing
your current pitta energies. This attraction to similar qualities may make it psychologically difficult to add opposite
qualities to your lifestyle when you wish to pacify a dosha.

Imagine, for instance, you have a number of vata-genic
factors (those that increase vata) in your lifestyle. These
may include living in a cold climate, having a job that
involves much travelling, especially flying, eating at irregular times, or habitually eating vata-aggravating foods (see

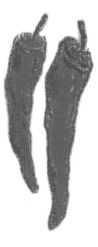

Chilli Peppers
*Chilli peppers increase the
pitta dosha, but pacify vata
and kapha. Your constitu-
tion, current doshic state,
and the seasons should all
be considered when decid-
ing if hot, spicy foods
should be part of your diet.*

Food Charts, pp. 132-43). These will increase your vata
energy until your vata dosha becomes excessive – unless
there are opposite qualities in your life. Lifestyle factors
that increase pitta include habitually eating salty or spicy
foods, or other foods that aggravate pitta; living in a hot
climate; or having a high-powered, competitive job. A
kapha-genic lifestyle could include over-eating, especially
foods that aggravate kapha, not exercising, sleeping excessively, and having a sedentary job.

Further, if your illness is due to an excess of the same
dosha as that predominating in your constitution, it is harder to treat. For example, a vata disorder (see p. 74 for examples) in someone with a vata constitution will be more difficult to control (as the constitution reinforces the disorder)
than in someone with a kapha constitution.

DOSHIC IMBALANCE ASSESSMENT

*When you have understood your constitution you can then determine if your doshas are in
balance. An imbalance is assessed by reading the signs and symptoms in your mind and
body that are manifested by the doshic energy that is excessive for YOU. If you have a persistent or chronic condition, complete this assessment in conjunction with the Ailment
Assessment on page 80.*

* *Repeat the physiological and psychological sections of the constitutional assessment (see
  pp. 38-41), to assess how you are NOW and have been recently. Differences in this and
  your original assessment indicate which dosha is excessive if the assessments have been
  done accurately.*
* *If you are experiencing any digestive discomforts, negative emotions, or sleeping
  problems, write down what you are experiencing and then relate their qualities to vata,
  pitta, and kapha, using the information on pages 30-1, 68-9, 75-7, 78, and 124.*

*This information will help you decide whether you are experiencing excess vata, pitta, or
kapha. If you are, you should look at your lifestyle (see Chapter 5) and diet (see Chapter 6)
to see what factors in your life are contributing to the imbalance. Then you can take steps to
restore your balance and prevent illness developing.*

FACTORS DISTURBING VPK

The ideal situation is to be able to read the doshas in your body, and live a life that maintains your constitutional balance. If circumstances, either external or internal, arise that cause an imbalance, the sooner you restore the balance the better. Ways to pacify the doshas will be discussed in Part Three, based on the principle that "opposites decrease".

Generally, it is an "excess" of a particular food, substance, activity, or emotion that will disturb a dosha, and so may start the disease process. What is excessive will vary from individual to individual, and will also vary for each individual at different times of his or her life. Your individual tolerances at any particular time are related to your constitution, the current state of your doshic energies, your age, and the season.

Increasing VPK
The table (opposite) lists frequent causes of disturbance to each dosha. Under the tenet of "like increases like" you may see why some aspects of your life increase your doshas. Generally, it is habitual excesses that aggravate the doshas. But if one of your doshas is already increased, then you may be intolerant even to small amounts of something with qualities similar to your increased dosha.

Place & climate
Traumas

Some Factors Affecting Wellbeing
All our experiences and circumstances have qualities and these can be related to the qualities of vata, pitta, and kapha. Those that have similar qualities to a dosha will increase it; those with dissimilar qualities will decrease it.

Age
Constitution
Season

Suppression of natural urges
Lifestyle
Occupation
Misuse of the mind, inappropriate actions and speech
Diet
Digestion & metabolism

Immunity
Misuse, or over or underuse of the senses
Mind & emotions

FACTORS THAT INCREASE VPK

VATA	PITTA	KAPHA
Exposure to cold	Exposure to heat	Exposure to cold
No routine in your life	Eating too much red meat, salt, spicy or sour foods	Eating too much sweet food, meat, fats, cheese, milk, ice cream, yoghurt, fried foods
Eating too much dry, frozen or left-over food, or foods with bitter, pungent or astringent tastes	Indigestion and irregularity of meals	Excessive use of salt
Fasting	Exercising at midday	Excessive intake of water
Too much travelling	Drugs, especially antibiotics	Eating after satisfaction
Too much or inappropriate exercise	Too much intellectual work/thinking	Taking naps after meals
Misuse/overuse of senses	Alcohol	Not exercising
Too much sex	Fatigue	Underuse of the senses
Alcohol	Anger, hate, fear of failure, and repression of these emotions	Too much sleep
Suppressing natural urges	Summer	Doing nothing
Abdominal surgery		Sedatives and tranquillizers
Stimulants and other drugs		Doubts, greed and possessiveness, lack of compassion and staying attached to these emotions
Too little sleep, staying up late, working nights		Late winter and spring
Not oiling the skin		
Frequent colonics/enemas		
Worry, fear, anxiety, grief – and repressing these		
Autumn and early winter		

INTESTINAL GASES

Gases indicate poor digestion and the formation of ama (p. 77); they prevent proper absorption of water, minerals, and prana in the colon. Associated mainly with excess vata, they may result from poor digestion due to derangement of any dosha. Their causes are mainly dietary, but they may also be due to inadequate sleep, nervousness, shock, worry, stress, or anger.

Advice for Preventing and Relieving Gases

• *Follow a diet suitable for your doshic needs and the rules of eating (see Chapter 6).*

• *Do not eat foods that are difficult to digest or that create gases in their digestion.*

• *Do not eat between meals, or too much at any meal, or too late at night.*

• *Leave at least three hours between meals to allow the stomach time to do its work.*

• *Avoid the sweet taste or only take small amounts on its own. Desserts after meals contribute to fermentation and gases.*

• *Use carminative (gas-dispelling) herbs in moderation when preparing foods (see pp. 158-9).*

• *For relieving gases, do knee-to-chest exercises (p. 127) and abdominal massage (p. 120).*

Habitual Suppression of Natural Urges

Charaka Samhita lists 13 natural urges and the symptoms that can occur if they are habitually suppressed (see italic text under each urge). Vata is the dosha that causes these urges and suppressing them disturbs vata. The symptoms are all therefore examples of disturbed vata. The symptoms, which may arise from habitual suppression of the natural urges, could be relieved by taking steps to pacify vata and by allowing expression of these urges in a manner that does not cause offence to other people.

URGE: URINATION

Possible symptoms
Pain in bladder and urethra, dysuria (painful or difficult urination), headache, stiffness in groin

URGE: PASSING GASES

Possible symptoms
Retention of feces, urine, and gases, flatulence, pain, exhaustion, and other disorders in abdomen due to vata imbalance

URGE: DEFECATION

Possible symptoms
Colic pain, headache, retention of gases and feces, cramps in calf muscles, and flatulence

URGE: EJACULATION OF SEMEN

Possible symptoms
Pain in penis and scrotum, body ache, pain in cardiac region, and obstruction in urine

URGE: YAWNING

Possible symptoms
Convulsion, numbness, tremors

URGE: SNEEZING

Possible symptoms
Stiffness of back of neck, headache, facial paralysis, migraine, and weakness of sense organs

URGE: VOMITING

Possible symptoms
Itching, urticarial rashes, anorexia, blackish spots on the face, swelling, anemia, skin diseases, nausea, and erysipelas

URGE: BURPING

Possible symptoms
*Hiccups, shortness of breath,
anorexia, tremors*

URGE: HUNGER

Possible symptoms
*Emaciation, weakness,
body ache, anorexia, gid-
diness, poor complexion*

URGE: THIRST

Possible symptoms
*Dryness of throat and mouth,
deafness, fatigue, depression,
cardiac pain*

URGE: STRONG BREATHING OR
PANTING DUE TO EXERCISE

Possible symptoms
Heart diseases and fainting

URGE: TEARS

Possible symptoms
*Coryza (catarrhal inflam-
mation of nasal mucous
membrane), eye diseases,
heart diseases, anorexia,
giddiness*

URGE: SLEEP

Possible symptoms
*Yawning, body ache, drowsiness, head
disorders, and heaviness in eyes*

Caution: *The above lists indicate the possible outcome of habitually suppressing your natural urges.
However, the symptoms may arise for other reasons.
Do not assume, for example, that all heart disease is
caused by not breathing properly after exercise.*

EARLY STAGES OF THE DISEASE PROCESS

According to Ayurveda an imbalance of the doshas lies behind all illness. An imbalance occurs when the current state of your doshas differs from your constitution. There are many ways in which the doshas can be disturbed (see pp. 64-5). A change or accumulation of a dosha may result from one primary cause, or from the cumulative effects of many causes. The cause may be strong and sudden (for example, receiving news of a sudden death), and have an immediate impact on the doshas.

More usually, the cause is weak and builds up slowly over time. It may come from an external source: eating an inappropriate diet over a number of years would, for example, cause a gradual change in the balance of the doshas. Or the cause of the disturbance of the doshas may come from within the body: for example, an accumulation of

Stage One:
Accumulation
The first stage is an increase in a dosha. The dosha accumulates in its seat, but at a rate faster than the body expels the excess. You may not notice the first signs of the disease process, since they are initially discomforts (see examples on chart opposite), and are not the sort of thing for which you are likely to seek therapeutic help. Many of us accept a modicum of discomfort as part of life or "my age".

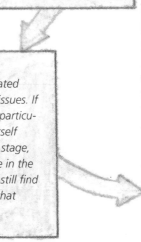

Stage Two: Provocation
If the accumulation is not stopped at Stage One, the excess dosha is provoked to leave its seat in the gastro-intestinal tract (see p. 46). The signs of an aggravated dosha become more noticeable (see p. 69).

Stage Three: Spread
In this stage, the aggravated dosha spreads into the tissues. If there is a weakness in a particu-lar tissue it will deposit itself there (see p. 70). At this stage, you may notice a change in the symptoms, but you may still find it difficult to pin-point what exactly is wrong.

If you pacify the excess dosha before the fourth stage of the disease process is reached (see p. 70), no lasting damage is done to the body. It is easier to regain your constitutional balance before the excess dosha settles into the tissues.

One, two, or all three of the doshas can be upset at any one time. Even where the initial difficulties arose from an excess of a single dosha, if left unchecked, the other two doshas are also likely to become disturbed in time. By then, a complicated illness will have developed.

toxins due to poor metabolism would impede the movement of vata and disturb the doshas (see also pp. 76-7). To
maintain wellness, observe and analyze your lifestyle to see
if you are accumulating too many qualities of a particular
dosha, and make any changes needed to balance your
doshas (see Chapter Eight).

Ayurveda describes the disease process in six stages.
The first three are described on these pages, the final three
on pages 70 and 72.

Chart of Signs and Symptoms
*The signs of the first three stages of
the disease process are grouped
according to which dosha is in excess
of its constitutional balance. You may
only have one of the symptoms on this
list; everyone has a different balance of
doshas at work in the body, and this
means that symptoms are different for
everybody. Remember – do not read
one symptom in isolation. Signs of
increased doshas are sometimes felt,
with the experience of negative
emotions (see p. 78).*

AGGRAVATED DOSHA	ACCUMULATION STAGE	PROVOCATION STAGE	SPREAD STAGE
EXCESS VATA	Constipation Intestinal gases Dry mouth Craves warmth Fear/anxiety	Increased gases & constipation Cold hands & feet Dryness in body	Distension relieved Fatigue Restless mind Worries/fear/anxious
EXCESS PITTA	Stomach acidity Burning sensations Anger/criticism	Heartburn Acid indigestion Burning pain in navel area Hypercritical	Burning sensation on passing urine/stools Yellowish stools Painful digestion
EXCESS KAPHA	Lethargic Low appetite Heaviness	Nausea Bloating Desire to sleep Increased salivation	Heaviness Swelling, Edema Increased mucus Vomiting

WEAK SPOTS

The fourth stage of the disease process starts when the spreading excess dosha finds a weak spot in one of the tissue types (see pp. 56-7), and settles there. The first warning signals of illness will be felt and, in the West, this is the point where we begin to feel that all is not well and take note of our lack of health. Through pulse diagnosis and a deep knowledge of the human body, an experienced Ayurvedic physician can read these warning signals and the earlier signs, and have a good indication of the disease that will follow if the excess dosha is left unchecked.

Weakness in Tissues
Weakness or defects in tissues arise from many causes, but can be classified as one of six types (below). Weak spots can be present in any part of the body, but symptoms from them only arise when an excess dosha has settled in the affected tissue.

Inherited Weak Spots
Asymptomatic weakness in the tissues arising from cellular memory of parents' and grandparents' illnesses.

Unresolved Emotions
Weakness in organs from unresolved or repressed emotions (see pp. 172-3).

Past Life Actions
In cultures that accept reincarnation, a weakness can be brought from previous lives. "Past life" also includes previous actions and attitudes in this life, and also a poor lifestyle.

Physical and Psychological Traumas
Tissues that have been physically damaged may retain a cellular memory of the trauma. Psychological trauma may weaken tissues. Certain negative emotions have an affinity to certain organs (see p. 172).

Previous Infections and Illnesses
A tissue is weakened when it is affected by disease, making it more vulnerable in the future.

Addictions
Tissues are damaged by addictions. Alcohol, for example, weakens the liver, smoking attacks the lungs, mind-altering drugs affect the brain, and an addiction to sex damages the genitals.

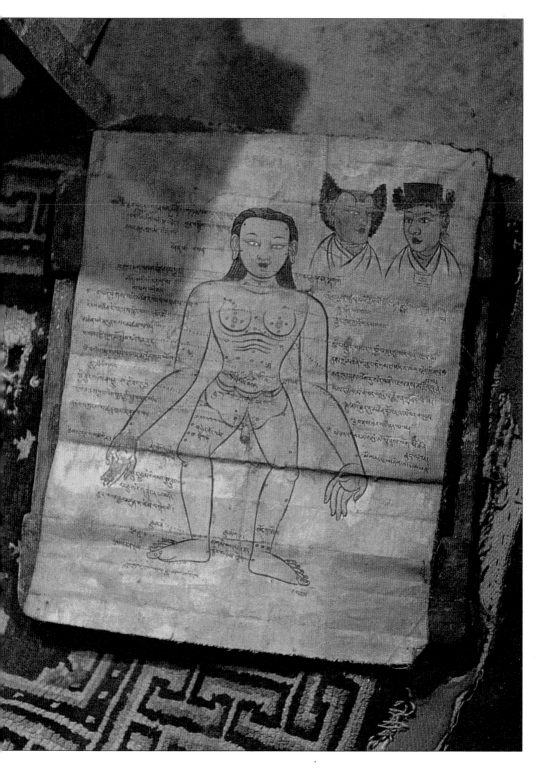

LATER STAGES OF THE DISEASE PROCESS

The fourth stage will only be reached if there is a weakness in one of the tissue types. If there is no such weakness, the excess dosha remains in circulation in the body, but causes no additional signs. Once Stage Five is reached, the disease needs rooting out and treatment is required. At Stage Six, the excess dosha will leave a weakness in the body and, unless pacified, will spread to other tissues.

Stage Four: Deposition
The excess dosha settles in the first tissue type that has a weakness. The dosha combines with the tissue, causing it, together with the by-products and "raw" materials, to become inferior. It may also produce toxins. If the tissue agni is strong, it will protect the tissue from the effects of an excess dosha.

Stage Five: Manifestation
At first, the effect of an excess dosha during deposition may be minor. But like a weed the disease grows and needs eradicating by eliminating the excess levels of the imbalanced dosha. Ayurvedic physicians may recommend panchakarma and/or herbs (see pp. 186-7) to restore the doshic balance. You should complement any treatment with changes to your diet or lifestyle to pacify the excess dosha and prevent recurrence of the illness.

Stage Six: Differentiation
The excess dosha has disrupted the integrity of the system and the disease and its complications can be named. The disease, like the perennial weed, may broadcast the seeds of future illness, or it may lie dormant only to grow again when conditions permit. Even if the excess dosha is pacified, a weakness remains in the body. If the dosha is not pacified, and only the symptoms ameliorated, the excess dosha may move and settle into other tissues, where further ramifications will ensue.

SIGNS WHEN DOSHAS ENTER TISSUES

When considering your ailments from the Ayurvedic point of view, try to think about the qualities of the signs and symptoms and relate these to vata, pitta, and kapha, and to the tissue types affected.

For instance, symptoms that have qualities of a mainly dry or degenerative nature are a result of imbalanced vata, as are those relating to underweight and loss of, or interference with, movement. Heat or inflammation qualities are connected with pitta, as is bleeding. Excess kapha is connected with being overweight, or other increases in body mass or excess fluids, such as tumours and swellings.

However, the story is not that simple, since the doshas also interact with each other. When this happens the experience of an Ayurvedic practitioner is required. A build-up of excessive kapha can, for example, block the free movement of the vata energy. Although impaired movement is the obvious symptom, kapha is at the root of it.

Dryness may be due to the heat of pitta drying the body. In this case, pitta, rather than vata, should be pacified. In making an assessment of doshic disturbances, Ayurvedic practitioners may trace the sequential pattern of disturbance from the order in which the symptoms arose.

Abnormal movements may arise because of problems with muscle or nerve tissue types. An Ayurvedic practitioner is trained to observe the interactions and know which tissues are disturbed by the excess doshas and how the doshas are interacting.

The table on page 74 is not comprehensive, yet it gives examples of how excess doshas may manifest in the seven tissue types. Symptoms should not be read in isolation but as part of an overall picture. In the West, words used to describe illness often involve one or more doshas or tissues, and do not class qualities separately. Eczema, for example, may be either dry or weeping, and Ayurveda says the root cause is different in each case.

SOME SIGNS OF DOSHA ENTRY INTO TISSUES

Tissue Type	Excess Dosha	Symptoms
Lymph	V	Cold hands and feet~Dehydration, dry skin~Sunken eyes~Tingling, numbness in the skin~Looks undernourished~Feels fear~Insecurity, anxiety, lack of confidence
	P	Fever~Acne, pimples~Hot flushes~Eyes sensitive to bright light~Critical, short tempered
	K	Retention of water~Indigestion~Loss of appetite~Lethargic~Colds~Bronchial congestion
Blood	V	Anemia~Dizziness~Abnormal pulsations~Contraction of blood vessels~Dry eczema
	P	Inflammatory conditions~Rashes~Fevers~Bruises easily~Nose bleeds~Bleeding under the skin~Psoriasis~Dermatitis ~ Multiple moles
	K	Weeping eczema~High cholesterol~Enlarged liver/spleen (dealing with excess fat)
Muscle	V	Muscle atrophy~Increased tone~Spasticity~Loss of movement~Tremors
	P	Repeated attacks of tonsillitis~Muscle abscess
	K	Muscle hypertrophy~Decreased tone, flabby muscles~Cysts on muscle tendons
Fat	V	Dry skin~Low back ache~Cracking of joints
	P	Profuse sweating~Cellulitis~Burning hands and feet~Burning sensation at tip of penis
	K	Excessive thirst~High cholesterol~Obesity~Thick white vaginal discharge
Bones	V	Hair loss~Brittle nails~Deformities of nails~Pain in the bones~Degenerative arthritis~Receding gums~Dental caries~Pain due to unresolved emotions
	P	Inflammatory arthritis~Bone abscesses
	K	Bone tumours
Nerve	V	Dizziness, fainting~Lack of co-ordination~Paralysis~Confusion~Loss of memory
	P	Paralysis~Multiple sclerosis~Aplastic anemia~Misunderstandings
	K	Tumours~Misconceptions
Reproductive tissue	V	Sexual debility~Low fertility~Premature ejaculation
	P	Inflammation of genitals
	K	Enlarged prostate~Tumours of testicles or ovaries/uterus

Pain

Vata is involved in all pain. If the vata flow of energy in the body is unobstructed there is no pain. Pain arises when the vata dosha is disturbed, or the flow of vata (the mobile dosha) is blocked by improper functions of pitta or kapha. Blockages may also be caused by accumulations of ama (see p. 77) or by the repression of emotions.

Repressed emotions can disturb the doshas and be the root cause of pain. Understanding such emotions can bring release (see p. 168).

Different Kinds of Pain
Ayurveda classifies pain according to the factor obstructing the flow of vata. The nature of the pain will reflect the qualities of this factor. Relate the qualities of your pain to the qualities of the doshas.

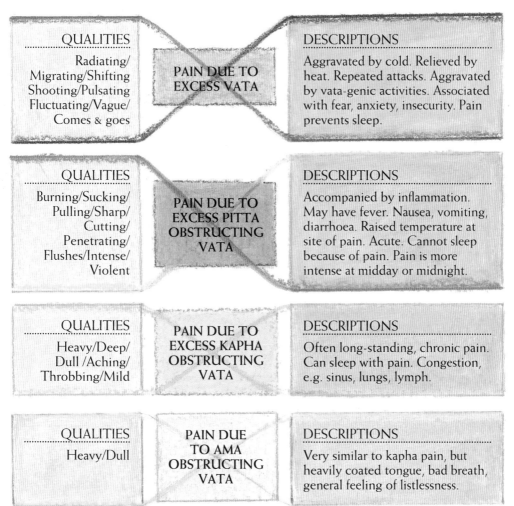

QUALITIES		DESCRIPTIONS
Radiating/ Migrating/Shifting Shooting/Pulsating Fluctuating/Vague/ Comes & goes	**PAIN DUE TO EXCESS VATA**	Aggravated by cold. Relieved by heat. Repeated attacks. Aggravated by vata-genic activities. Associated with fear, anxiety, insecurity. Pain prevents sleep.
QUALITIES		DESCRIPTIONS
Burning/Sucking/ Pulling/Sharp/ Cutting/ Penetrating/ Flushes/Intense/ Violent	**PAIN DUE TO EXCESS PITTA OBSTRUCTING VATA**	Accompanied by inflammation. May have fever. Nausea, vomiting, diarrhoea. Raised temperature at site of pain. Acute. Cannot sleep because of pain. Pain is more intense at midday or midnight.
QUALITIES		DESCRIPTIONS
Heavy/Deep/ Dull /Aching/ Throbbing/Mild	**PAIN DUE TO EXCESS KAPHA OBSTRUCTING VATA**	Often long-standing, chronic pain. Can sleep with pain. Congestion, e.g. sinus, lungs, lymph.
QUALITIES		DESCRIPTIONS
Heavy/Dull	**PAIN DUE TO AMA OBSTRUCTING VATA**	Very similar to kapha pain, but heavily coated tongue, bad breath, general feeling of listlessness.

Disturbed Metabolism

An imbalance of doshas can disturb agni and metabolism (see p. 48) and will impair your ability to digest food. If agni is low, toxic substances called *ama* (see p. 77) are produced. The body is not always able to expel ama, in which case it is deposited in various parts of the body, blocking or interfering with the free flow of dense and subtle matter through the body's channels.

This is especially so in the case of the digestion agni. For example, chyle – the form food becomes as it is absorbed through the intestine walls – may contain partially digested food. Although this may be absorbed, partially digested food fails to provide, or inhibits the use of, nutrients needed by the body.

Disturbed Digestive Agni
Ayurveda describes indigestion according to which excess dosha is affecting agni. The symptoms of poor digestion reflect the qualities of the imbalanced dosha. All three types of poor digestion produce ama.

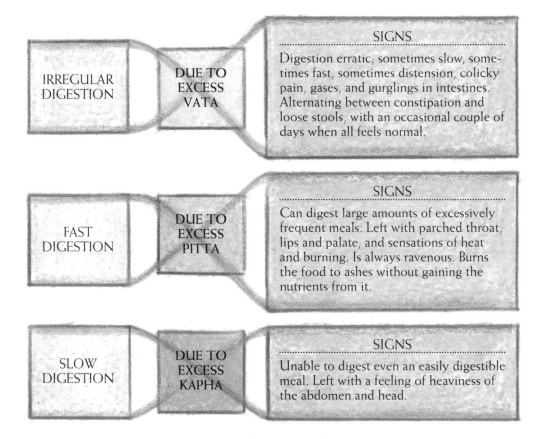

IRREGULAR DIGESTION

DUE TO EXCESS VATA

SIGNS

Digestion erratic; sometimes slow, sometimes fast, sometimes distension, colicky pain, gases, and gurglings in intestines. Alternating between constipation and loose stools, with an occasional couple of days when all feels normal.

FAST DIGESTION

DUE TO EXCESS PITTA

SIGNS

Can digest large amounts of excessively frequent meals. Left with parched throat, lips and palate, and sensations of heat and burning. Is always ravenous. Burns the food to ashes without gaining the nutrients from it.

SLOW DIGESTION

DUE TO EXCESS KAPHA

SIGNS

Unable to digest even an easily digestible meal. Left with a feeling of heaviness of the abdomen and head.

Derangements of agni and the production of ama are internal causes of disease. Deranged agni disturbs the doshas and
also increases the production of ama. This will disturb agni
still further, setting up vicious circles of cause and effect. The
main causes of disturbed agni are:
- doshic imbalance
- excessive eating or drinking
- prolonged fasting
- eating between meals
- repressed emotions (see pp. 170-3)
- ignoring the rules of eating (see p. 154), but especially
  - wrong food combinations
  - foods inappropriate for your constitution
  - eating at unsuitable times
  - eating heavy, frozen, cold, or spoilt food
- improper use of purgatives or laxatives.
   If the tissue agnis (see pp. 56-7) are defective, inferior
tissues and their by-products will result. Other effects of
defective tissue agni are to lessen the body's ability to
produce ojas (see p. 56) and to protect the tissues from the
effects of excess doshas (see p. 72).

AMA

*Ayurveda considers ama to be a major cause of illness. The Sanskrit word encom-
passes toxins in the body, whether these were originally external poisons
introduced into the body or ones created internally due to low agni, poor food
combinations, inadequate elimination of wastes, or disturbed doshas. Some of the
literal meanings of ama include raw, uncooked, immature, and undigested.*

*A defective tissue agni will also result in ama during the production of the seven
tissues (pp. 56-7). A subtle ama is produced if our mental processes are impaired,
or if we harbour unresolved emotions (see Chapter 7).*

*A whitish coating over the whole tongue indicates ama throughout the body. If
the back third of the tongue is coated there is ama in the colon. If the coating is
brownish, vata is disturbed as well. Bad breath and body odour are other signs of
ama in the body. Ayurvedic physicians often recommend herbs to eliminate ama
and balance agni.*

NEGATIVE EMOTIONS

A doshic imbalance may have a negative effect on your mind and emotions. If a dosha is in excess you are more likely to display negative energy of a quality associated with it. The predominant dosha of your constitution becomes excessive more easily than the others. Thus, you will tend to experience its negative aspects more than others.

Negative emotions aggravate the dosha associated with them. For example, high kapha may mean you are more possessive but possessiveness increases kapha. The way to break this vicious circle is to pacify the aggravated dosha.

Thinking in qualities and using Ayurveda in your daily life will help you to become more conscious of the qualities of your moods and to rate these as V, P, and/or K. This is a useful way to monitor small increases in a dosha, and to take steps to restore the balance sooner rather than later. Relate the qualities of your moods to the qualities in other aspects of your life. Remember "like increases like". If you are impatient or critical (pitta), check if you have eaten pitta-genic foods or been exposed to pitta-provoking experiences.

Negative States
This lists below classify negative emotional and mental states according to excess doshas. By referring to the lists on pp. 30-1 and the positive states (see Chapter 7), you can compare how excess doshic energy may affect your mind and feelings.

EXCESS VATA
Nervousness ~ Anxiety ~ Fear ~ Confusion ~ Grief ~ Sadness ~ Insecurity ~ Lack of Integrity ~ Loss of creativity ~ Lack of communication ~ Moodiness

EXCESS PITTA
Ambition ~ Anger ~ Envy ~ Fear of Failure ~ Frustration ~ Hate ~ Jealousy ~ Judgmental or critical tendencies ~ Snappy speech and actions ~ Lack of discernment ~ Pride ~ Scepticism

EXCESS KAPHA
Boredom ~ Carelessness ~ Lack of compassion ~ Greed ~ Feeling lack of support or love ~ Obsessive behaviour ~ Unkindness ~ Lack of interest

AILMENTS

The Ayurvedic concept of the disease process is difficult to grasp initially, since it challenges how we have been taught in the West. As we have seen, symptoms of ill health can be classified into vata, pitta, and kapha, and this will indicate which dosha is likely to need pacifying (see table on page 74). Sometimes, the idea may seem too simple to be credible, and at others too complex to master. This is a natural reaction of the mind to new ideas. As you observe your life and body in terms of doshas you will see these concepts working in practice.

The first stages of the disease process deal with minor ailments that can be ameliorated by knowing yourself, and making appropriate adjustments to your lifestyle. The ability to read the initial signs of imbalances is the key to regaining wellness.

In the latter stages of the disease process the balance between your doshas, tissues, and agni has been seriously disturbed, and often complicated further by the presence of ama. You should seek qualified help in these stages, but lifestyle and diet are still important to support any treatments undertaken.

Symptoms of PMS
When you are assessing any ailment from the Ayurvedic perspective, it is important to look at the qualities of each symptom and classify them according to VPK. The name given to your ailment is not the key factor as the illness may be due to a disturbance of any one of the doshas. The symptoms of PMS are well known, and are related to VPK in the lists below.

VATA

Bloated belly

Low back ache

Painful joints

Stiffness and tightness in muscles

Insecurity, anxiety, fear

Irregular menses, with scanty flow

PITTA

Hot flushes

Red, sensitive eyes

Nipples sensitive to touch

Burning sensation in urethra

Burning sensation in hands and feet

Migraine headache

Anger, criticism

Argumentative

KAPHA

Retention of water

Breasts enlarged and full and tender

Gains weight

Tiredness, excess sleep, lethargy

Craves/eats sweet taste, especially chocolate

Very possessive

Heavy flow

AILMENT ASSESSMENT

The interactions of the doshas in the body are complex.
Give yourself time first to learn the qualities each dosha
may manifest (see pp. 30-1) and also to understand your
constitution (see pp. 38-41). Then you can start to appreciate if any excess doshic energy is affecting you. Remember,
skilful reading of the doshas in the body comes with practice. As your knowledge of Ayurveda increases you will
make more accurate assessments of your doshic state.
But initially focus on your most intense, persistent, or
chronic symptom or ailment. First, assess your doshic
imbalance (p. 63). Then describe the ailment you are experiencing and answer these questions to help you grasp the
qualities in your ailment and to relate them to VPK:

• *What predominant qualities are you experiencing?*
• *Describe the quality of the pain, if any (see p. 75)*
• *When did the symptoms begin? In which age (see p. 10),*
  season (see p. 150), and climate?
• *Do your symptoms change with the seasons, climates, or at dif-*
  ferent times of the day or night (see p. 151)?
• *Did you experience any major life events before the symptoms*
  began (see p. 170)?
• *What steps have you taken to alleviate the symptoms? What*
  qualities did these measures have? What effects did the alleviat-
  ing steps have?

See pages 30-1 and this chapter to help you decide if an
excess of VPK is causing your symptoms. Remember to
seek the advice of your medical adviser if you have an
ailment or illness.

   Maintaining good health is an ongoing process. The
more you practice thinking in qualities and about
Ayurveda, the more you will refine your perspective about
your condition and learn how much emphasis to give to
the variety of factors. At the same time, you will improve
the way you adjust your diet and lifestyle to maintain your
doshas in balance. If this balance is restored, you will have
no excess dosha to cause symptoms of ill health.

AYURVEDIC PROFILE: GILES
Age: 30
Height: 6ft. 4ins.
Weight: 210 lbs.
Constitution: Kapha, with pitta as secondary dosha

Find out more
about Giles
on pages 156-7.

After finishing school, Giles took a desk job, ate a diet of junk food, did his fair share of drinking, smoked, and indulged in recreational drugs. At 22, he married and became a student for three years. He reduced his alcohol intake and only smoked and took drugs under stress. He continued eating a diet rich in dairy, sweet, and fried foods. On completing his studies, he joined a personnel department where he still works. Five years ago, his grand-father – with whom he had been close – died. His wife left him a year ago and he still feels the pain of desertion.

As a child, Giles caught mumps, measles, and whoop-ing cough but has had no major illnesses since. For some years, he has suffered congestion of the nasal sinuses, which is worse in winter and spring. He often has cold hands and recently has been drinking more fluids and urinating more often.

A year ago, Giles started coughing, expelling thick mucus from his lungs. The expectoration is worse in the evenings. He likes plenty of sleep and he sleeps deeply. He often feels very heavy after eating. His bowel movements are regular but slow, and his stools are soft and sticky with some mucus.

Interpretation: The ailments that Giles is experiencing have kapha characteristics – obstruction, coldness, heavi-ness, excess mucus, and a desire for more fluids. The drinking, smoking, and drugs may have caused weak spots in his liver, lungs, and brain respectively.

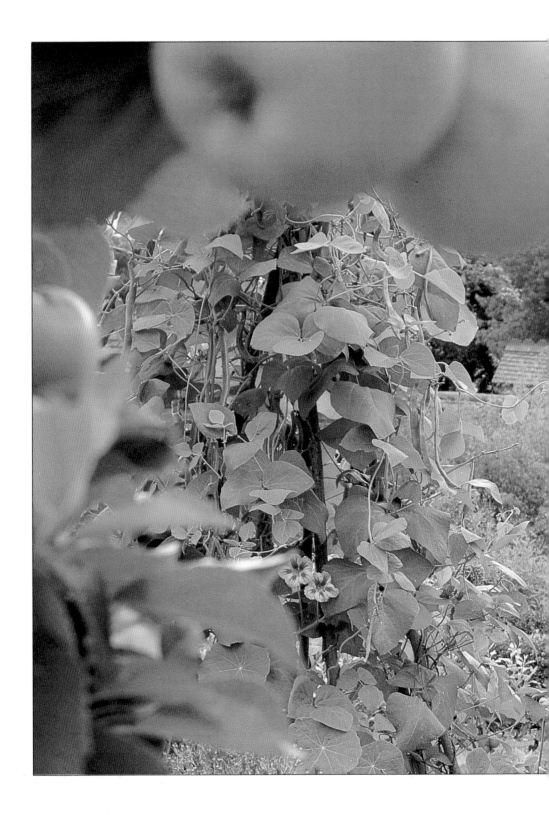

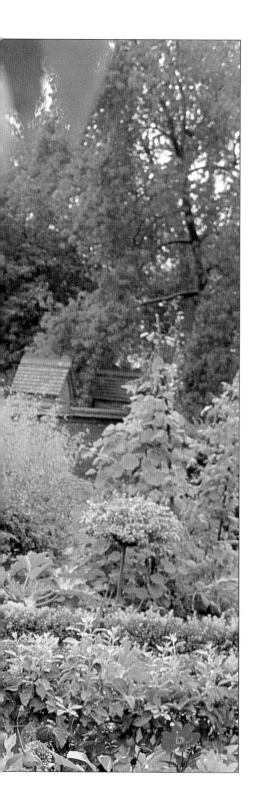

PART THREE

Maintaining Wellness

Daily Activities

तस्याशिताद्याद्याहाराद्बलं वर्णश्च वर्धते ।
यस्यर्तुसात्म्यं विदितं चेष्टाहारव्यपाश्रयम् ॥

He, who indulges daily in healthy foods and activities, who discriminates (the good and bad of everything and then acts wisely), who is not attached (too much), to the objects of the senses, who develops the habit of charity, of considering all as equal (requiring kindness), of truthfulness, of pardoning and keeping company of good persons only, becomes free from all diseases. (**Astanga Hrdayam** *Chapter 4: 36*)

Everything we do has particular doshic characteristics. The way we eat, sleep, work, and enjoy ourselves – all have qualities of VPK. It is important to realize that everyone can adjust their personal daily routine to redress a doshic imbalance and maximize wellbeing. If, however, you continue to behave in ways that increase any imbalance in your doshas, you will not experience the satisfaction of a high level of wellbeing. A sustained imbalance in your doshas will lead to illness.

Achieving a doshic balance does not happen overnight – you have to work at it. The best way to start is to ask yourself questions about how you lead your life. Truthful answers will begin the process of raising your awareness, which will guide any adjustments you then decide to make. Remember that change has to come from you. Other people's suggestions can only help you if you have truly accepted the changes that you are trying to bring about.

Some of your daily activities are more fixed than others. The nature of your work, for example, may be difficult to change, whereas you can design leisure activities to counteract the excessive influence of a particular dosha. Use your exercise and leisure activities as opportunities to counter any imbalances that arise from your working patterns (see pp. 88-91), and allow yourself time to nurture your mental, emotional, and inner aspects.

Some of the guidelines in the pages that follow apply to everyone. Others are intended to adjust specific doshic imbalances. This chapter provides basic routines that can help you balance your doshas. It may require great effort to change established habits, but once you notice the small benefits of initial changes you can move from a downward spiral of ill health to an upward path of wellness.

The way of Ayurveda is to look at changing the balance of all activities, not to try to tackle symptoms in isolation. If you make general changes in your life that are right for you, your doshic balance will improve so that, when you no longer have excess doshic energy, many symptoms you might have will disappear of their own accord.

TELEVISION

Watching too much television increases vata due to overstimulation of the eyes and ears. It also increases kapha due to the passive nature of watching. The subject matter watched may also affect the doshas. In Ayurveda, the principle of "like increases like" is important; for example, if the overall quality of a program has negative pitta emotions (see p. 78), these may be impressed on a subtle level on the mind, and may then increase pitta. If and how these subtle impressions manifest themselves in an individual depends on many factors, but it is unlikely that a direct correlation is possible. Habitually listening to fearful news bulletins may increase your vata levels. Be selective in your viewing and listening so you can take in only those subtle qualities you would like to have.

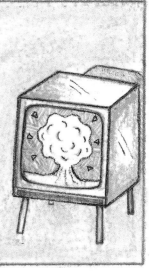

Daily Routine

Give a little thought to your daily routine and arrange the events of your life for your optimum wellbeing. Ask yourself whether your commitments, habits, and preferences are benefitting or disturbing your doshic balance. Modern pressures can make you feel that you have little choice over many aspects of your life. Yet, the accumulated benefits of small changes can make a noticeable difference to you.

Your constitution will influence the way you arrange your life. Read the following guidelines to see whether your approach to daily routine is helping you keep your doshas balanced, or whether you need to make adjustments to help prevent increases of your predominant dosha.

Your Routine
A routine that is balanced for your constitutional type will allow you to enjoy freshness and vitality every day.

PITTA

Pitta types may have already organized themselves efficiently – and often those around them, too. You tend to be precise about following your plans, as this helps you achieve your objectives. Avoid becoming too goal oriented. Take time to do things just for the sake of doing them – take a relaxing walk instead of playing a competitive game. Sitting outside on a clear summer's night staring at the moon is very soothing for pitta.

VATA

Vata types need to introduce regularity to their lives and keep it – one of the hardest things for a vata person to achieve. But in succeeding you will experience less erratic levels of energy and a decrease in the discomforts caused by excess vata, such as insomnia and weariness. Eat regularly and establish a routine for going to bed and getting up.

Keep your routine even when your energy is good. Note when you are running on overdrive – unable to pay enough attention to your current task, frantically doing three things at once, or talking fast and frequently, skipping from subject to subject. Slow down and give yourself time to think; you will still achieve all you need to, but will be less tired.

KAPHA

If you already have a fixed schedule and don't like change, you are probably a kapha type. Review your routine often, making deliberate changes to prevent yourself from getting stuck in a rut. Overcome your kapha dislike of change by making a pact with yourself to do something in a slightly different way each day – for example, vary your route to work.

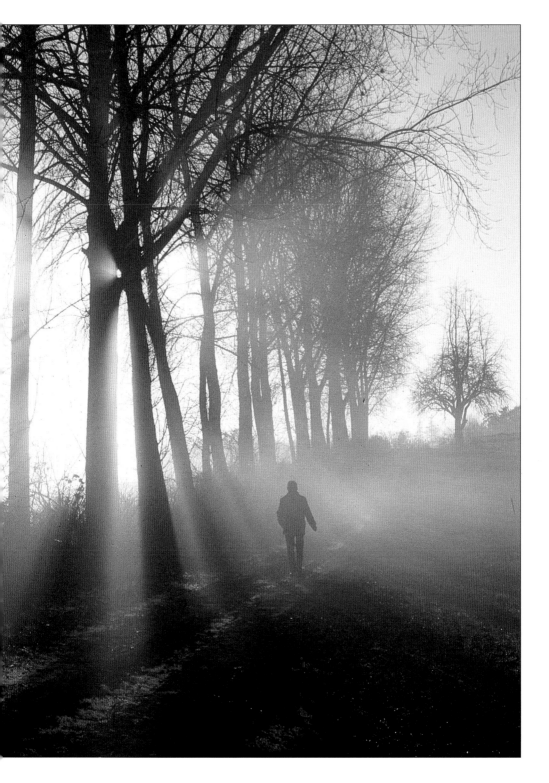

VPK AT WORK

You may spend as much as a third of your day working, so the many qualities associated with your work and working environment will affect your doshas. If your assessments (see pp. 104-5) show that the accumulated effects of work result in a steady increase of one or more doshas, then you may have to adjust your diet, daily routine, and leisure pursuits to balance it.

The qualities of different occupations can be related to the qualities of vata, pitta, and kapha (see right). Bear these qualities in mind when recruiting others and look for someone with a good balance of the necessary qualities in their constitution. However, if in excess these doshic qualities will manifest themselves as negative characteristics. For example, a reliable administrator (kapha) may be unwilling to accept change if her kapha increases excessively. Similarly, the efficient manager (pitta) may concentrate on his or her personal objectives rather than company ones, and the creative designer (vata) may have unworkable ideas.

Much tension arises when you have to work with someone who evokes strong emotions in you. These will also affect your doshas (see p. 78). Reflect on these difficulties in your quiet times to tease out the different levels in the problem and why you react as you do. Look deeply, but without being hard on yourself. Try to understand the situation, without attributing fault. You may find ways of resolving the problem. It may not be easy to change the outer circumstances but you can limit the detrimental effects on your wellbeing by becoming an "observer" (see Chapter Seven).

When considering the effect of work on your doshas, you need to take into account the qualities of your working environment. There may be subtle psychological influences. For example, the threat of redundancy brings with it a fear of unemployment and change, which increases vata; or competitiveness, instead of co-operation with your colleagues, increases pitta.

Constitutional Suitability

The chart on the right shows examples of occupations related to the qualities of vata, pitta, and kapha (VPK). The airy qualities of vata are good for communication skills; the ether element adds creativity. A strong intellect is associated with pitta; so too is the precision exhibited, for example, by competent engineers. The steadiness and compassion of kapha is appreciated in the caring professions, and the earth element in kapha finds good expression in horticulture and catering. Inevitably, many occupations call on qualities from all doshas.

OCCUPATIONAL VPK

VATA	PITTA	KAPHA
Dancing	Management	Nursing
Acting	Politics	Administration
Designing	Surgery	Cooking
Teaching	Law	Building
Writing	Finance	Counselling
Photography		Manual labour

The Working Environment

Using the examples in the chart below, try to relate the qualities of your working environment to vata, pitta, and kapha.

EFFECT OF WORKING ENVIRONMENT ON DOSHAS

ENVIRONMENT	CONDITIONS	INCREASED DOSHA
Air-conditioned office or department store	Lack of prana in atmosphere Lack of natural light Flickering artificial light	Vata Kapha or Vata Vata
Airplane	Movement, lack of prana, dehydration	Vata
Car/truck	Movement	Vata
Kitchen	Heat	Pitta
Furnace, foundry	Heat	Pitta
Cold store	Cold	Vata and Kapha
Check-out near exit door	Noise and draughts	Vata

Excess experience	Increases
Boredom	Kapha or vata
Challenges	Pitta; also vata, if they evoke fear
Competition	Pitta
Concentration	Pitta
Decision making	Pitta
Frustrations	Pitta
Interruptions	Vata
Repetitive tasks	Kapha
Small repetitive task involving the same muscle action	Vata
Responsibility	Pitta; also vata, if you worry about it
Sitting/standing	Kapha
Talking	Vata
Telephoning	Vata

Qualities at Work

Arrange the qualities of your work environment to help you keep your doshas balanced. Try to have natural light and ventilation, freedom from intrusive noise, the right space and a pleasing décor.

The Nature of your Work

When you assess any detrimental effects your work has on your doshas, consider those qualities that become excessive. Study the table (left) and the effects that an excessive experience can have on the doshas.

COMPUTERS

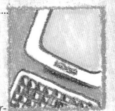

Computers have become part of modern life, in both the work place and at home. Some of their adverse effects are now known, and guidelines have been laid down for working practices to limit adverse influences on health. If you spend too much time working or playing with a computer it will increase all three doshas, but especially vata. The speed at which the information on the screen changes, the flickering of the screen (often subliminal), and the repetitive sensory and motor stimulation all disturb vata. The precision needed, and the many frustrations that arise in obtaining the required results, increase pitta. Eye strain can disturb both vata and pitta. The sedentary nature and repetitive routine of computer work increase kapha.

Take steps to pacify vata by massaging your face, hands, and forearms with oil. Take frequent breaks away from your computer, preferably in fresh air; and move and stretch your body frequently, in particular the fingers, hands, arms, and shoulders. Spend a few minutes, two or three times a day, resting your eyes. One way to do this is to rest your elbows on your desk or your knees, close your eyes, and cover them with your palms.

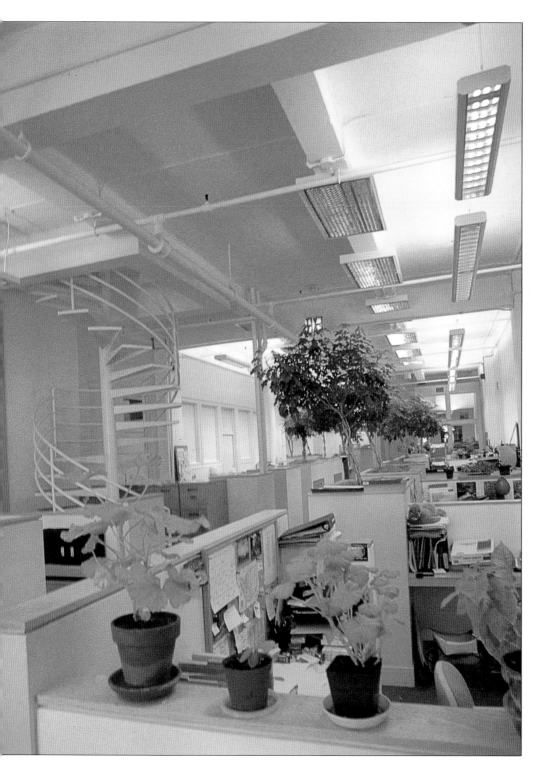

LEISURE PURSUITS

By understanding the qualities associated with your leisure activities you will, in the short term, be able to add opposite qualities to reduce some of the adverse effects caused, for example, by your working life. Choose activities for relaxation and leisure to suit your constitution and so lead to balance and harmony in your life. For example, gentle, soft music will soothe vata, but kaphas may need the stimulation of louder, livelier music.

Consider the long-term consequences of your leisure pursuits on your doshas – you may be having fun now, but are you building up trouble for the future? For instance, you may enjoy being very active in your twenties and thirties, but could overstep the fine line between a healthy level of activity, which varies for each individual, and being slightly hyperactive. Hyperactivity increases vata energy. If the increase is gradual, you may not notice the effects until you are in your forties or fifties, by which time the excess dosha has moved into the deep tissues (see pp. 68-74).

Leisure Choice
Look at the doshic guidelines below to help you choose leisure activities appropriate to your constitution.

PITTA

Pittas are attracted to competitive, mentally challenging situations. You should be challenged enough to avoid the risk of boredom, but not in ways that make you aggressive or increase your determination to win. You should avoid competitive one-to-one contests.

VATA

Vata is easily increased by misuse or overuse of the senses, since vata predominates in the nervous system. Very loud music, fast flashing lights, and computer games, all overuse the senses. If you have a vata constitution you are naturally drawn to fast action and new experiences, but you should spend time doing calm, gentle, creative pursuits, such as painting and spinning. You will also benefit from saunas, because of their warm and moist qualities.

KAPHA

If allowed to, kaphas enjoy sitting doing nothing, whereas you would be better taking part in activities that are both physically and mentally stimulating. Make a concerted effort to take on new activities, but do not let these degenerate into unconscious habits. Keep adding variations to your leisure pursuits – for example, devise new aerobic sequences regularly.

Sports and Pastimes

If you frequently engage in sports, select those with qualities that help you balance the doshic qualities of your other activities, particularly your work. The table is given as a guide to help you relate sports and their various qualities to vata, pitta, and kapha. Remember that "like increases like". For example, engaging in vata-genic sport will increase your vata dosha. The way in which you play a sport may also alter the qualities. For example, if you are aggressive, this will increase pitta, as will competitiveness. Movement, speed, and action are vata qualities, and will therefore increase vata.

KAPHA
Angling~Bowls
Weightlifting~Wrestling
Shot putt

PITTA
Archery~Chess~Fencing
Shooting

VATA/PITTA
Football~Motor racing
Squash~Table tennis
Tennis~Track sports
Horse racing

VATA/KAPHA
Sailing~Windsurfing

PITTA/KAPHA
Billiards~Snooker~Golf
Javelin throwing~Boxing

VATA
Bobsledding~Bungee-jumping
Cycling~Gymnastics
Horse riding~Ice skating
Parachuting~Roller skating
Skiing

GARDENING

Gardening benefits all the doshas. It helps bring vatas down to earth, unless they are overly enthusiastic and exhaust themselves. Planning and the challenge of growing new varieties of plants or old ones more productively will keep pittas stimulated. Kaphas have an affinity with the land, and benefit from the physical work of gardening. The fresh air will also give extra prana which balances all the doshas.

On Vacation

Vacations give you a chance to have a change of scene, a break from your commitments, and time to relax once you arrive at your destination. All types of travel, especially flying, increase vata. Anxiety about flying also increases vata, making you even more anxious. Take steps to pacify vata on your journey. Avoid alcohol, since it adds to the dehydration, drink dilute sweet fruit juices instead; drink ginger tea or take ginger tablets; massage your face and hands with a light oil, perhaps with one drop of lavender essential oil per 5 ml (1 teaspoon) of base oil; and eat small, easily digestible meals.

A Change of Scene
Backpacking in snow-covered mountains is strenuous and challenging. It makes a suitable vacation if you have a pitta constitution, but it is not so good for vata types.

Choosing a Vacation
The type of vacation you take will affect your doshas. Select a vacation that has the right qualities to help balance your lifestyle.

VATA

If you have a vata constitution you will be most affected by change and new experiences. Sightseeing and touring are vata-genic. You would benefit most by having a vacation in a single destination with plenty of sun and warmth, though not in an arid climate. You will find locations at sea level less vata-aggravating than those at altitude. Resist packing your days and nights full of activities that leave you feeling tired. Find a beautiful place and enjoy being idle.

PITTA

If you have a pitta constitution avoid hot climates. Be sufficiently active to keep your mind satisfied by challenging yourself, rather than others. Try activities such as backpacking, canoeing, or skiing. Aim to let your holiday unfold and do not organize it to such an extent that you become frustrated if things do not go as planned.

KAPHA

If kapha predominates in your constitution, you may be most contented lying in the sun doing as little as possible. However, a touring or activity vacation, which brings new interests each day, would be more beneficial for you.

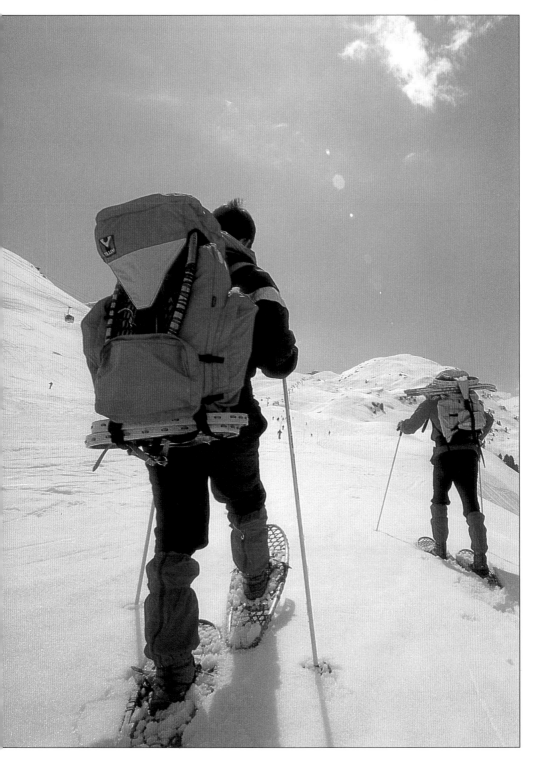

TAKING EXERCISE

Regular exercise helps improve the digestion: it raises agni, keeps the channels unobstructed, expels the wastes of cell metabolism, and keeps the muscles supple. Almost everyone will benefit from exercise, but the exercise must be suitable for your constitution. Too much exercise increases vata.

The ideal amount of exercise varies with each individual. Ayurveda says you should exercise to half your capacity. For instance, if you know that after running for thirty minutes you are exhausted, then you should not run for more than fifteen minutes. Another way to tell when you have had the optimum amount of exercise is when sweat comes to your forehead, armpits, and along your spine.

Exercise and VPK
Read the following guidelines to help you determine the best exercise for your constitution.

VATA

If you have a vata constitution, you are attracted to vigorous exercise, such as aerobics or jogging, and you often exercise to the point of exhaustion. However, exercising to this level increases vata, and in the long run will have a damaging effect on your joints, which are particularly vulnerable in people with a vata constitution. Have a regular amount of gentle exercise every day.

PITTA

If you have a pitta constitution, you should resist competitive sports such as tennis or squash. Your determination to win may cause you to take the sport too seriously. Water and winter sports will cool the heat of your pitta constitution.

KAPHA

If you have a kapha constitution, you may dislike exercising. You would benefit from vigorous exercise, though you may need a lot of encouragement to do so, until it is established as part of your routine. You will have the stamina to exercise for longer than those with a vata constitution.

Yoga, walking, and swimming are good exercise for all constitutional types, balancing for all three doshas, and can be
done alone or with others. If you are a vata type use your
enthusiasm to start a new exercise programme to encourage
one of your kapha friends to join you. A weekly arrangement for you and your kapha friend to meet together at the
swimming pool or yoga class will help you sustain the habit
when your initial excitement wears off. Your pitta friend
might join you once he sees how he will benefit.

Receiving a massage is a passive form of exercise, giving
the physiological benefits of exercise. It also helps counteract the stresses of modern life, particularly if you can lie
down for an hour in a pleasant and relaxing atmosphere
and let someone give you their full and caring attention.
Incorporate a regular weekly, fortnightly, or monthly
massage into your lifestyle in order to experience the
accumulating benefits.

Exercise need not be limited to times when you have an
hour to spare. Small amounts of exercise throughout the
day are beneficial. A short walk after eating will aid digestion. Get into the habit of stretching and relaxing different
muscle groups occasionally, especially if you have to sit for
long periods of time. Stretching or warm-up exercises first
thing in the morning balance the somnolence of the night.
Such exercises can also be done at any other time of the
day, but not after eating.

Caution: Do not take
strenuous exercise if you
have acute indigestion,
chest complaints, infec-
tions or inflammatory
complaints, or if you are
very old or very young.

SIMPLE EXERCISE SEQUENCE

Before you begin the exercises, sit still in the kneeling position (see right). Attune to your breathing, taking several deep, rhythmic abdominal breaths – let your abdominal muscles expand as you inhale and gently contract as you exhale. As you perform the sequence of exercises remain aware of your breathing and try to co-ordinate your movements with your breath.

When you first try these exercises do them slowly, taking one or two inhalations and exhalations in each position before moving to the next. Be aware of the stretching and contraction of your muscles. Do not strain in any way. Then sit in the kneeling position and, still maintaining the deep rhythmic abdominal breathing, picture your body performing the sequence of exercises. You can do this by visualizing the movements or imagining the feelings in your body, particularly your muscles, as you do them. Then repeat the exercises.

When you are familiar with the exercises, practise them daily to help keep your body flexible. Start with three rounds of the sequence and slowly increase to ten. It is important to remember that, before starting each sequence, to attune to your breathing since this will affect the speed at which you do the exercises.

When you are familiar with the exercises and are able to perform them with ease, you can do the sequence as a more dynamic exercise, especially if you have a kapha constitution, but remember to keep the co-ordination of breath and movement. When you have finished the sequence, remain for a few moments in the kneeling position – physically relaxed and mentally calm – and observe your breath.

The Kneeling Position
Kneel down, with your knees and heels slightly apart, but with your big toes touching. Then sit back so that your buttocks sit comfortably on your heels, hands resting on your thighs just above the knees. Check that your spine is straight but relaxed and your chin level so your neck and head feel aligned with your spine.

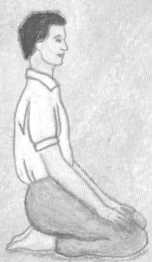

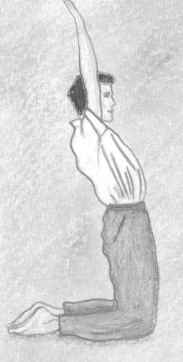

1 The Upward Stretch
Inhaling, remain kneeling, and simultaneously raise your buttocks and stretch your arms up in line with your ears, palms forward and fingers pointing to the ceiling.

2 The Resting Position
Exhaling, bend forward, bringing your forehead, hands (slightly apart), and elbows (bent) to rest on the floor, with your buttocks resting on your heels.

3 All-fours Position

Inhaling, without moving the position of the hands and knees, raise yourself to kneeling on all fours, with chin and buttocks up. Drop your abdomen and small of the back toward the floor to create a smooth curve in the lumbar area.

4a Preparation

Prepare to move into the inverted-V position by tucking your toes under, but remaining on all fours.

4b Inverted-V Position

Exhaling, push into the floor with your hands, straighten your legs so your buttocks go high into the air making your body into an inverted-V shape; put your head between your arms, aiming the crown of your head at the floor, and feel that your back and shoulders are flat. Place your heels flat on the floor, but do not force them.

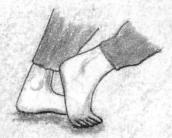

Note

If your heels do not easily go flat in the inverted-V position, practise walking on the spot by alternately bending one knee forward as the opposite heel goes down on the floor. Keep your toes on the floor as you do this.

5 Return to All-fours

Inhaling, return to the all-fours position.

6 Return to Resting

Exhaling, return to the resting position.

7 Back Stretch

Inhaling, slide your arms straight out in front, come on to your knees, move forward with your body, dropping your hips and buttocks toward the floor. Keep your arms straight so your body weight is held on the heels of your palms of the hands. Keep your chin up and look up.

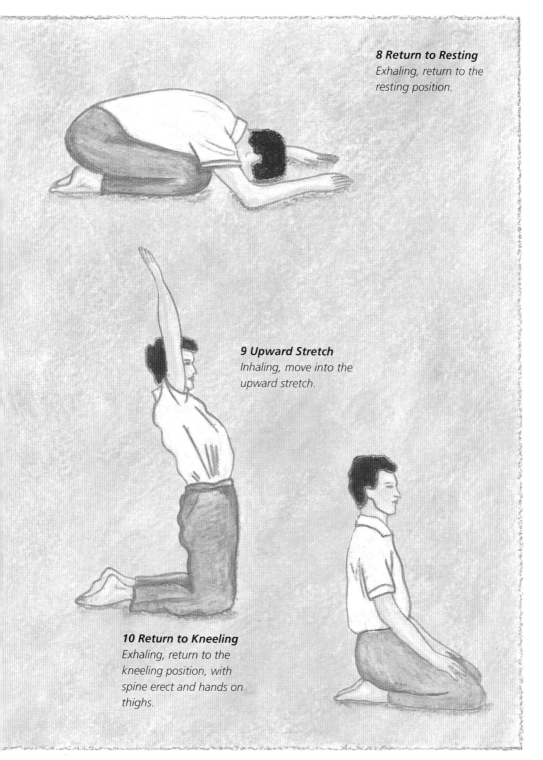

8 Return to Resting
Exhaling, return to the resting position.

9 Upward Stretch
Inhaling, move into the upward stretch.

10 Return to Kneeling
Exhaling, return to the kneeling position, with spine erect and hands on thighs.

WORK, LEISURE, AND EXERCISE ASSESSMENT

As you assess the doshic qualities of your work or your main daily activities you have to consider the strength of their influence, which may change from time to time. The overriding qualities of your office job may increase kapha, but if a new boss tries to undermine you or give you new responsibilities, that is likely to increase vata and pitta, too.

Use the list of questions (below and right) to start your work and leisure assessment. Write qualitative descriptions of all aspects of your work. Then, using the lists of qualities (see pp. 28-31 and 88-91), assess the effect your work has on your doshas. Ask which aspects need to be balanced, either by changing your working habits (if this is possible) or by altering other areas of your life, to bring overall doshic harmony. Consider also how much exercise you do and what you do in your leisure time. Look at the qualities to see the relationship between what you do and the doshas. Is this the right way for you to spend your time?

Work Assessment Questions

- *What skills do you use in your job?*
- *What intellectual, physical, and emotional demands are made on you while you are working?*
- *What is your working environment like?*
- *Does your job require you to sit or stand in a particular posture, or to hold or use part of your body in a particular way over long periods of time?*
- *What are the small experiences that you encounter day in and day out in your job?*
- *How much time do you spend working at a computer?*
- *How do you feel about your work?*
- *Are there any difficult relationships connected with your work?*

Leisure and Exercise Assessment Questions
- *How much leisure time do you have in a day/week?*
- *What exercise do you take? Is it too much or not enough?*
- *What sports do you play? How do your mind and body feel during and after sport?*
- *What are your hobbies and pastimes? What intellectual, physical, and emotional experiences are involved? What are their qualities?*
- *Do you experience any discomforts before, during, or after your leisure time, such as headaches or weariness?*
- *Do you watch television, listen to music? What other sensory experiences do you have?*
- *Do you regularly spend time, however short, with your partner, children, or friends?*

AYURVEDIC PROFILE: MARTIN
Age: 45
Height: 1.79m (5ft 10in)
Weight: 70.5kg (155 lbs)
Constitution: Pitta

Find out more about Martin on pages 156-7 and 182-3.

An ambitious lawyer described by his friends as a workaholic, Martin expects unrealistic standards from his employees. He makes fast decisions, hates failure, and has a quick temper. He can skip meals when engrossed in work, but this makes him very critical and when he stops work he is ravenous. He enjoys Italian and very hot Mexican foods. He plays squash and likes fast cars. He experiences acid indigestion and frequently has red spots and blotches on his face and neck. Once or twice a year, he gets a mild lung infection. Over the last year, he has had occasional but intense headaches.

Interpretation: *Martin is experiencing pitta ailments. His pitta constitution makes him intellectually capable and ambitious, but excess pitta drives him too hard. He fears failing so does not allow himself to ease up or to listen to advice until his body can no longer take the strain. His work and leisure activities are pitta-increasing.*

MORNING ROUTINE

Your body readily adapts itself to your habits, so it is important that you establish a routine that contributes to improving your overall health and vitality. Good habits often seem the most difficult to acquire. Your mind may resist change or may tell you that you are missing out on some of life's pleasures. But following a few simple guidelines (see pp. 108-9) for a short time each day – this may only involve thinking about something in a different way – is preferable to times of discomfort and illness that may affect you for longer periods.

Your current morning routine will probably have evolved to take into account the needs of getting to work on time and/or getting children up and off to school. You may feel that there is no time in the morning to do anything new or different. Introducing change may mean doing things in a slightly different way or getting up earlier (see pp. 112-13). If you decide to introduce changes to your morning habits, choose one or two alterations at first and gradually build up to a healthier routine

Early morning is the main vata time (see p. 151). Vata energy in the pelvic cavity is responsible for expelling urine and feces. Ayurveda teaches that the natural urge for defecation should arise in the early morning soon after naturally waking from sleep. As well as proper elimination, other important parts of the daily routine include stretching, or exercise (see pp. 96-103), and a few moments watching the breath. Together, these prepare the body and mind for a fresh intake of nutrients and experiences.

Morning Exercise
Regular stretching and gentle exercise as part of your morning routine help to regulate your body's metabolism.

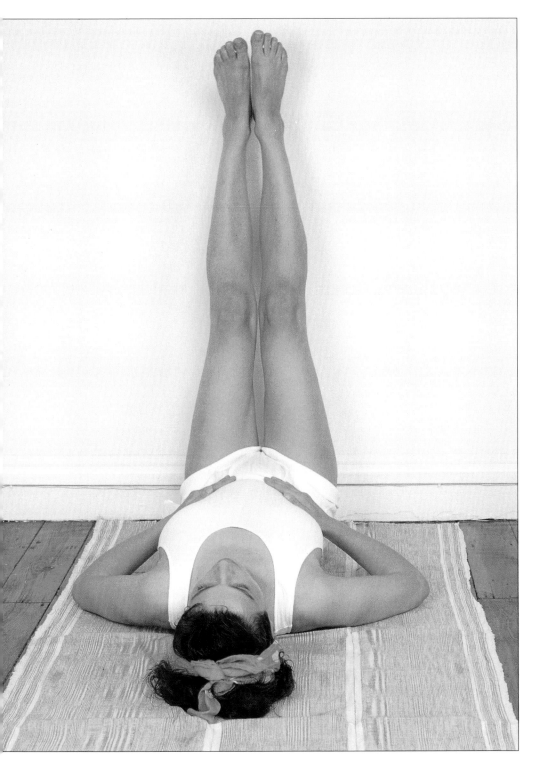

SUGGESTIONS FOR A MORNING ROUTINE

The following suggestions for a morning routine are suitable for all constitutional types. Use the suggestions to decide how you wish to alter your morning routine.

1 *On waking, lie in bed for a few moments and become aware of how your body is feeling, and of your attitude toward the new day. Think about all levels of your being, and your part in universal creation. Whatever the difficulties or challenges you may face during the day, start it with kind and loving thoughts about yourself. Adopt an attitude of thanks; this will keep your heart open to the wonder of the universe and its blessings. Try and carry this attitude of awareness into all your daily activities.*

2 *Rub your palms together and hold or gently rub them over your face before getting out of bed. Feel energy and vitality flowing into your being.*

3 *Greet yourself in the mirror, a reminder that you love and respect yourself.*

4 *Visit the bathroom and attend to the natural urges of elimination, which should arise in the morning (see pp. 126-7).*

5 *Gently scrape your tongue with a tongue scraper or teaspoon. This simulates the digestive system through subtle channels (similar to meridians) that connect with the tongue. If you have ama (see p. 77) in your body you may have a coated tongue and scraping it will help remove some of this.*

9 *Take a hot or warm shower or bath. Use only warm water on your head.*

8 *Oil your skin (see p 117).*

7 *Clean your nasal passages. Hold one nostril as you clear the other using deep abdominal breaths. Do not use short, shallow, or forceful breaths. Using your little finger, carefully massage each nostril with sesame oil, this will help prevent the mucus membranes drying. Your fingernail must be kept short if you do this.*

10 *Do some stretching exercises (see pp. 98-103) or yoga. And follow this with meditation or a quiet time.*

6 *Clean your teeth. If you have receding gums, massage them with your forefinger after dipping it in sesame oil. Repeat this in the evening.*

11 *Dress in fresh, clean, comfortable clothes. Select colours according to their effects on your doshas (see pp. 110-11).*

12 *Eat breakfast, if it is appropriate for your constitution (see p. 151).*

THE EFFECTS OF COLOUR

Different qualities are associated with different colours. You can relate the colours to vata, pitta, and kapha and use colour to affect your wellbeing, particularly through the colours you choose for your clothes and the decor of your home and work place.

The range of hues reflects the different facets of a colour. For example, red is associated with heat, violence, aggression, passion, power, domination, but it can also be stimulating, warming, and comforting.

YELLOW AND ORANGE
Yellow and orange are warm, stimulating colours that increase pitta. Their strong, dark shades are not advised if you have a pitta constitution or high pitta dosha, but sunny yellows will cheer vatas who are prone to depression.

RED
Red will over-stimulate pitta, but can be warming for vata, and provide necessary stimulation for kapha. Pink is gentler, embracing, loving, and calming, but if you have a kapha constitution it may make you more lethargic. Red cars are not to be recommended, as they could add a touch too much aggression to your driving, especially if you have a pitta constitution.

GREEN
Green with a yellow hue will increase pitta and decrease vata. Blue-greens will cool and calm pitta, and increase kapha.

GOLD

Gold, the colour of the sun, is warming, and can be used if you have a vata or kapha constitution. Silver is connected with the moon and is cooling. If you have a pitta constitution you could perhaps wear silver jewellery rather than gold.

BLUE AND PURPLE

Blue and purple are cooling colours that can be worn to good effect by those with pitta constitutions.

CONSTITUTIONAL TIPS

Each constitutional type should ideally decorate their home in colours that pacify their predominant dosha. Vata's homes should be in warm pastel colours; pitta's in cool blues and greens; kapha's with bright designs and colours.

Kapha Avoid using white if you are a kapha. All colours pacify kapha, except greens and dark blues. Choose bright, strong, bold colours and designs that will excite you.

Vata If you are a vata type, blue and other dark shades probably predominate in your wardrobe. Ideally, you should avoid dark colours, especially black, browns, and blues. You should also avoid vivid colours which may disturb the sensitivity of the nervous vata. Choose pastel shades instead.

Pitta Eliminate red and black from your wardrobe if you are a pitta type. Use cool, soft, pale colours and blues as much as possible.

MORNING ASSESSMENT

Few of us look in detail at our experiences between waking and starting the day's main activities. List the things you do in the morning and in what order you do them (see below). Add how you feel when you awake and your attitude to starting the day. Compare your list to the suggested routine on pages 108-9 to see if you need to make adjustments. What changes would you like to make (for example, get up 20 minutes earlier to do stretching exercises or sit down to eat breakfast) and what do you need to make them happen?

If part of your schedule involves getting your child up and off to school, include in your assessment what you do for your child, and any feelings and frustrations you have. Do you wish to adapt some of these habits and attitudes as your child's ability to care for him or herself increases?

The following questions can help you become aware of your morning habits – are they right for your doshas?

- *What time do you wake up? Does it allow you enough time to prepare for the day without rushing?*
- *How long do you lie in bed before you get up? What do you think about? Are you looking forward to a new day?*
- *Do you get the urge to eliminate your bowel and bladder first thing in the morning? Do you attend to them? Are two or three bowel movements necessary? Do you need to drink tea or coffee to stimulate a bowel movement?*
- *How many cups of tea, coffee, or other drinks do you have in the morning?*
- *Is your skin dry? Do you oil it regularly or apply drying products, such as talc or alcohol-based perfumes?*
- *Do you stretch or exercise your body?*
- *Do you meditate or take time to compose your thoughts?*
- *Is the television or radio on? Is it background noise or are you paying attention to it?*
- *Do you eat breakfast, and if so at what time? Do you sit down or eat as you go?*
- *How do you feel by the time you are ready to start your day's pursuits?*

AYURVEDIC PROFILE: VICKY
Age: 60
Height: 1.61m (5ft 3in)
Weight: 48kg (105lbs)
Constitution: Vata

Find out more about Vicky on page 156.

Vicky retired 6 months ago. Although she has had no serious illness, for most of her life she has suffered frequent indigestion, variable appetite, gases, and alternating bouts of constipation and loose stools. She has dry skin, a dry cough, and often feels cold, especially her feet. She sleeps fitfully, and most of the time feels weary. Recently, she noticed tics in her hands and fingers.

Vicky has a general anxiety that does not allow her to relax. She has a coated tongue and often has bad breath. She has little routine in her life, going to bed at any time between 8 pm and midnight depending on how she feels. Occasionally, she takes a walk. She says she takes no other exercise as she is always running around. Her mind jumps from idea to idea and she starts more projects than she will ever finish.

Interpretation: Vicky is experiencing ailments due to an excess of vata energy, enhanced by the changes brought on by retirement. The bad breath and coating on the tongue indicate toxins, perhaps due to poor digestion resulting from increased vata and poor food combinations. Vicky will find it hard to get into and stick with a daily routine, yet this is the best way for her to pacify her vata.

Vicky is establishing a new morning routine. She rises at 6.30 am and attends to elimination, which is becoming regular since she started taking triphala (see pp. 128-9) each evening. She applies sesame oil before showering, and cleans her mouth and nasal passages. Since joining a weekly yoga class Vicky practises for half an hour with a 10-minute breathing and quiet time at the end. At 7.45 am, she eats breakfast.

Since retiring, Vicky has looked at the colours of her clothes. When shopping, she is still drawn to blue, her favourite colour, but has decided to add pink and beige. She could also try warm reds, especially in winter.

HOMECOMING

Late afternoon and early evening are vata times. For many people, this is the time to leave work, to travel home, and to change their activities. It is easy to take this diurnal increase in vata energy into your evening. As soon as you get home, shower, change into fresh clothes, and have 10 minutes' quiet time. Use this time to detach yourself from the day's events and remind yourself "who you really are" (see Chapter Seven).

Try not to take your concerns about work home with you. If you do, make a mental effort to put them to one side, until it is the appropriate time to deal with them again. At the same time, ask yourself to be receptive to the guidance of your intuition in your decisions and actions regarding your concerns. It may take practice before this works well for you, but sincerity and persistence will be rewarded.

You can also use the quiet time to connect with your inner wisdom regarding conflicts and difficulties in your domestic life. If your household arrangements, or the need to prepare the evening meal, make it difficult to take a few quiet moments, remember that it is your conscious attitude that really makes the difference and that you are never separated from your inner wisdom.

Eat your evening meal early to allow time for the food to digest before engaging in other activities. You should leave at least two hours between eating and going to bed.

Spend some time with your children, your partner, your friends, or with yourself each evening, without modern distractions, such as the telephone or television. Give your attention to the moment, unfettered by your regrets from the past or your concerns about the future. Tiredness can make you irritable and snappy in company, but by really listening to each other, and by allowing time and space for acceptance, you will be able to foster spontaneity and understanding.

Inner Tranquillity
Take a few moments at the end of your working day to close your eyes and contact your inner beauty and peace.

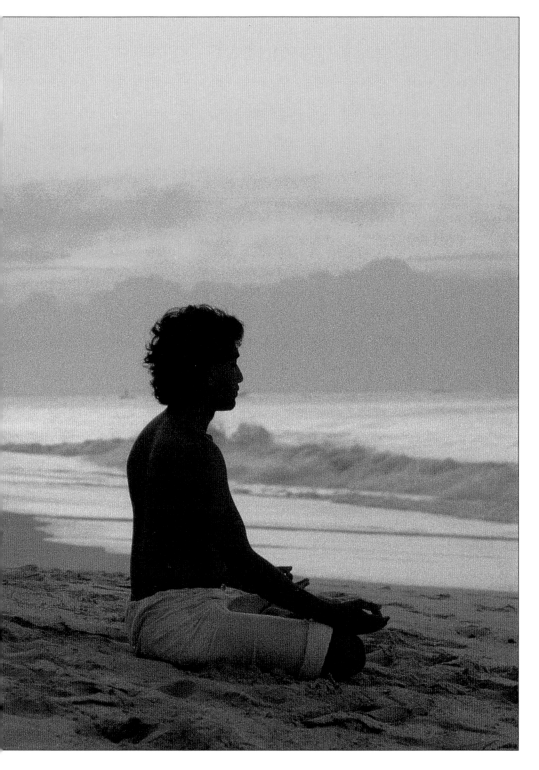

INTIMACY

The natural time for intimacy is during kapha time in the evening, as the sexual act increases vata due to the amount of energy expended throughout the mind and body.

Satisfying sexual union between two people brings increased health, vitality, ojas (see p. 56), and thus immunity. It has to be developed over time, with each partner being concerned most with their partner's satisfaction on physical, mental, emotional, and deep inner levels. Thus, they build up a trust that allows the surrender of the defences of their innermost being, allowing each to open completely to the other and the unity of orgasm.

Reciprocal satisfaction cannot be hurried and needs a certain propriety. Though touch and smell are the primary senses of intimacy, every sense should be satisfied. Intimacy needs pleasant surroundings – flowers, soft music, sweet foods. Bathe in warm water perfumed with oils. Healthy sex also needs the clarity of total awareness (see pp. 176-7).

Gratification of lust and unsatisfying sex will bring ill health due to increased doshas, loss of ojas, and thus reduced immunity. Excessive loss of reproductive tissue weakens other tissue types and this is aggravated by dryness in the cells from increased vata. Unsatisfying sex also disturbs the emotions, and thus the doshas, principally pitta from anger and frustration, but also vata if fear or vulnerability is experienced, or kapha if you are possessive.

Desire to gratify lust may lead to an addiction to sex and frequent changing of partners in vain attempts to reach the deep satisfaction that can be found in sexual union. Vatas may change their partners because they seek satisfaction through new experiences; pittas in search of an intensity they cannot, or feel unable to, achieve; and kaphas because, once interested in sex, they have big appetites.

The frequency of sex depends on your constitution and also the seasons – it is more depleting in hot weather than cold. Kaphas have greater stamina and are able to partake more frequently and for longer than vatas and pittas.

REPRODUCTIVE TISSUES

Milk, honey, ghee, and onions are nourishing foods for the reproductive tissues. But onions arouse the body, which could cause further sexual desire. Warm milk with honey and almonds is advised after sex to help replenish the tissues.

OILING

Regularly oiling the skin keeps it smooth and supple. It is a very useful way to pacify vata, counteract dryness, and reduce anxiety. If you have a vata constitution or are in the vata age (see p. 10), try to oil yourself at least three times a week. A weekly oiling of the whole body is recommended for everyone (unless there are contra-indications).

Sesame oil is favoured in Ayurveda. It is warming and heavy and very pacifying for vata. Kapha is naturally oily and those with increased kapha should use oils very sparingly. Sesame oil may be too heating for pittas; sunflower or coconut would be more suitable. Use organic, cold-pressed oils; these are available from wholefood shops.

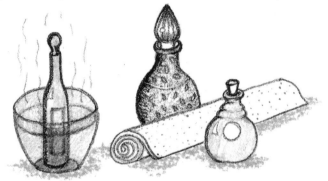

Contra-indications

Do not use oil:

- If you have a medical condition or are pregnant, unless with the consent and knowledge of your medical adviser.
- Over any areas that are painful, unless you have guidance from your medical adviser or a massage therapist.
- Over any areas of broken, damaged, or infected skin.
- Within an hour of eating.
- If you have a thick coat on your tongue, an indication of ama.

Tips about Using Oil

- Oil, especially sesame oil, is very penetrating and difficult to remove from fabrics, particularly man-made ones. Do not use your best towels, keep one specifically for use when oiling up. Put on cotton socks after oiling your feet to protect carpets and bedding.
- Do not put oil on the soles of your feet if you are going to bathe or shower afterward since they will be slippery. Take care in the shower or bath since any excess oil on your body may leave a film on the bath. Clean the bath immediately.
- Warm oil is comforting and penetrates the skin better than cold oil.
- If you have long hair and find it difficult to get the oil on to your scalp, use a small dropper filled with oil and run the tip along your scalp slowly releasing the oil. Then massage.
- Keep oil in a small bottle with a nozzle to help control the amount used.
- Warm the oil by putting the bottle in a bowl of warm water.
- Keep paper towels to hand for wiping your hands and any spills immediately.

Instructions for Oiling

- *Have an attitude of nurturing and love toward yourself and your body. Keep your attention on the part of your body you are oiling.*
- *Sit or stand on a large towel spread on the floor in a warm place.*
- *Use small amounts of oil, adding more as it is absorbed. Using both hands and adapting to the contours of your body, work in generous circular movements and long strokes from the extremities toward the body. Vatas should be gentle with themselves but kaphas can be more vigorous.*

Massaging the Scalp

A sense of calmness and tranquillity comes from massaging your scalp with oil. Such a massage pacifies vata and can reduce feelings of general anxiety.

Oiling Head and Feet

A shorter method of applying oil, which can be used at night to bring calmness and aid sleep, is to apply oil to your head and feet. Apply oil to the crown of your head and massage for a few moments with your fingertips. If you do not like getting oil on your hair, apply it to the forehead and temples instead. (A towel over your pillow will help protect it from oil.) Sitting on the floor, apply oil to the soles of your feet and massage them for a minute or so. Put on cotton socks.

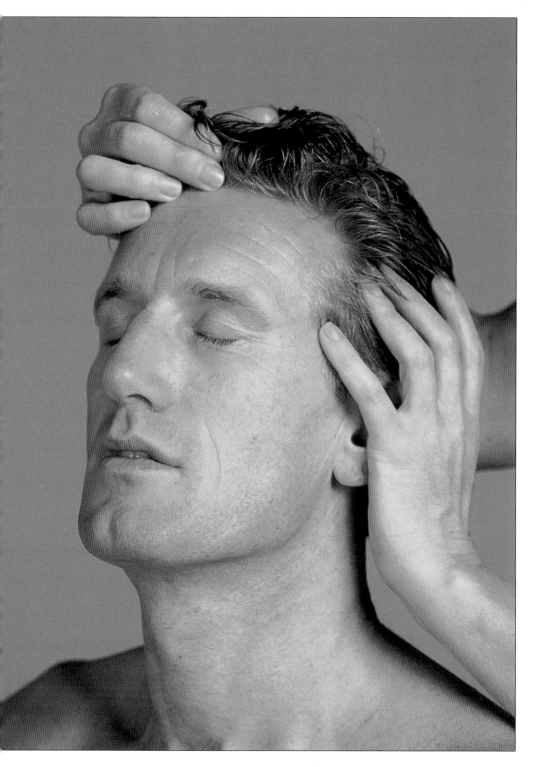

Sequence for Oiling

- Work oil into your fingers, thumbs, and hands.
- Work up both arms to your shoulders and into your armpits.
- Apply oil to your toes, especially around the nails, and then work over the tops of your feet and up your legs.

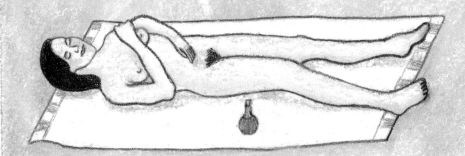

- A very comfortable way to oil your abdomen is to lie on your back on the floor with your knees bent and your feet flat on the floor. However, you can do it sitting or standing. Place one hand flat on your abdomen and put the other over it. Work in the direction of flow in the colon: come up your right side to your rib cage, across your middle, down to your left hip, and across to your right hip.

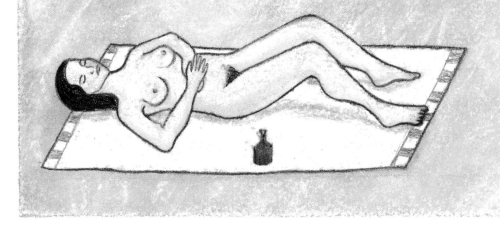

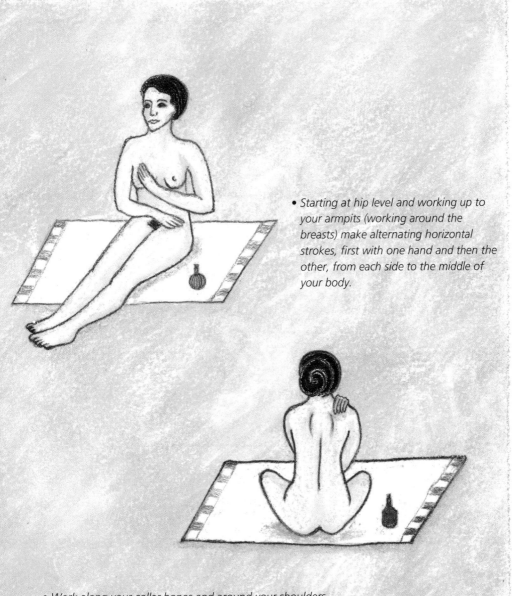

• Starting at hip level and working up to your armpits (working around the breasts) make alternating horizontal strokes, first with one hand and then the other, from each side to the middle of your body.

• Work along your collar bones and around your shoulders.
• Using your fingers work up and down the back of the neck, and more gently at the front.
• Using your fingertips work gently, but firmly, over your face (avoiding your eyes). Also, oil your scalp if you wish.
• Only oil those parts of your back that you can reach easily.
• Shower or bathe after you have finished.

OILING WITH A FRIEND

It can be very relaxing to have someone apply the oil for you. This person can be a partner or a friend whom you can trust. They do not need to oil your whole body, just your back, or head and feet, or your face.

Sit or lie in a comfortable position – this will depend on which parts of your body are to be oiled. As you relax, your body temperature naturally drops a little so it is important that only the part being massaged is uncovered. Feeling chilled will prevent you from relaxing. And make sure your "oiling friend" has warm hands. Give your friend feedback about the pressure they are applying – whether it is too light or too heavy, or if it is just right.

Getting Ready

Make sure your "oiling friend" is comfortable, to avoid a stressed back through bad posture. If you lie down, use a massage table or the floor. Avoid using a bed, if possible, as it offers you little support and the height will almost certainly be wrong for your partner. Remember, your partner's clothes need to be protected from the oil by using a towel either as an apron or placed on their lap if massaging your hand.

Your "oiling friend" should use circular strokes to work the oil into your skin with their fingers or hands, depending on the area being oiled.

For the Vata Age
Oiling is very beneficial to counteract the dryness experienced in the vata age (over 55). Many who are well into the vata age will enjoy having oil rubbed gently into their hands. One drop of lavender essential oil per 5 ml (one teaspoon) of base oil will give added comfort.

SLEEP AND DREAMS

Evening is kapha time, which brings a natural heaviness to your mind and body. The main requirement for a good night's sleep is the complete digestion of all the day's mental and emotional experiences, and also of food.

Too much sleep increases kapha. Kaphas and those with excess kapha should avoid sleeping during the day or having a lie-in. Vatas need plenty of rest to replenish their nervous system and should avoid late nights and night shifts. Pittas sleep soundly, generally require less sleep than other doshic types, and usually wake with an alert mind.

Sleep problems can be related to the doshas. Going to sleep easily but having difficulty waking can indicate excess kapha. Waking around midnight relates to increased pitta. Difficulty going to sleep, waking frequently – especially between 2 and 4 am – indicates that your vata is too high.

If you find it hard to go to sleep, train your mind and body to accept that going to bed means going to sleep. Set a time for going to bed, preferably between 10 and 11 pm. Massage your head and feet with sesame oil (see p. 118). Drink a cup of milk (see pp. 160-1). If you are taking triphala (see pp. 128-9) in the evening, you need to alter your routine: take the triphala at least an hour and a half after eating and a milk drink at least an hour and a half after the triphala.

A Pleasant Bedroom
Use fresh bed linen, soft lighting, and gentle music. Do not have a television or reading matter by the bed, other than perhaps a book of inspirational quotes.

Dreams

During sleep, the mind withdraws the senses from the outer world. It has the opportunity to finish digesting the day's experiences and completing unfulfilled desires. When you remember your dreams you may be recalling fragments of these processes.

Dreams can be related to the doshas. Vata dreams are either active with movement, such as flying, chases, jumping or falling from heights, or are frightening. Pitta dreams can be violent or angry, or have sharp instruments or fighting in them. Kapha dreams are gentle, often featuring calm water, lakes, or oceans.

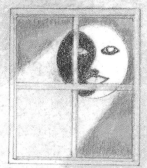

Your dreams will tend to relate to your predominant dosha (see pp. 38-41). A change in the type of dreams you have may indicate a doshic imbalance (see p. 62). For example, if you start experiencing dreams with vata qualities, they may indicate an increase in your vata dosha.

Occasionally, you may have a dream that seems significant to you. Trust yourself to interpret it. Ask yourself questions about the people, objects, situations, and relationships in the dream. Be guided by your inner wisdom as you enquire, remaining open in order to gain the insights that will be useful to you.

Sequence to Combat Insomnia

- Sit on your bed and watch your breath for a few moments, give thanks for the day's experiences, joys, and tribulations.
- Get into bed, put the light out.
- Still watching your breath get into a position that is comfortable for sleeping. If you are restless, just know that it is your excess vata energy wanting to fidget.
- Stay watching your breathing. Imagine what your body feels like when it is asleep. Let your breath slowly deepen. Repeat this exercise if you wake in the night. Often insomnia makes us feel that we will be tired the next day, but by doing this exercise you can ensure that your body at least will be rested.

CONSTIPATION

The colon is the seat of vata (see p. 46), and an important organ for the overall wellbeing of the body. It is part
of the food and prana channels: an unhealthy colon
means that elimination and digestion may be impaired
and absorption of prana from food reduced. In addition,
toxins may be assimilated into the body, and vata could
increase, possibly leading to excess vata spreading to
other parts of the body.

Chronic constipation tends to be connected with
increased vata, but may be due to an increase in the
other doshas. The excess heat of pitta may cause dry
stools. The downward movement of the vata energy,
which is responsible for defecation, may be blocked by
too much mucus in the intestines (increased kapha) or by
an accumulation of undigested foods or ama.

An inappropriate diet with poor food combinations is
a major cause of chronic constipation and gases. Lack of
sleep, anxiety, and other factors that increase vata (see
p. 65) may also contribute to constipation and gases.
Habitually suppressing the natural urge for defecation, or
the excessive use of laxatives or colonics may also result
in constipation, since they all upset the body's natural
intelligence to regulate itself.

Early morning is the vata time of day and the
best time for elimination. Waking around 6 am
to attend to the natural urges of defecation
with complete and satisfying elimination
helps to maintain the health of your colon.

The Squatting Position
*Stand with your feet hip-
width apart and toes turned
outward. Bend the knees
and slowly ease yourself
down as far as you can comfortably go. Practise moving
up and down until you can
squat comfortably.
Eventually, you will be able
to wrap your arms around
your knees and hug them.
This position may take many
weeks of practice. Do not
force this position, and if it
becomes uncomfortable,
release it.*

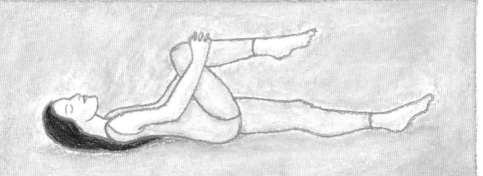

Knee-to-chest Exercises

1 Lie on the floor and bend your right knee. Hold your leg just below the knee and pull it toward your abdomen (below). Release your leg and return it to the floor. Repeat with the other leg.

2 Lie on the floor and bring both knees up simultaneously. Wrap your arms around your legs, just below your knees, and hug them (above). Pull them in toward your abdomen. Hold for a few moments. Relax and return your legs to the floor. Try to do this exercise twice a day.

Some Ways to Help Relieve Chronic Constipation

- *Check your diet, especially for inappropriate food combinations and excess of vata-genic foods (see the NO column of food charts – pp. 133-43). Check other factors that may be disturbing your doshas and slowly make changes in your diet and lifestyle.*
- *Condition your colon to regular elimination. On rising, go to the bathroom, even if you do not have the urge to defecate. Sit or squat (see below), pull in your anal muscles firmly, and relax. Repeat three times. Don't push or strain as you try to pass stools.*
- *Drink a glass of warm water to help stimulate the gastro-intestinal reflex.*
- *Take triphala before going to bed (see pp. 128-9).*
- *Practise squatting twice a day (see left), and if possible use this position instead of sitting when passing stools as it aids complete elimination.*
- *Do the knee-to-chest exercise twice a day.*
- *Massage the abdomen (see p. 120) with or without oil. If you cannot easily fit this into your daily routine, do it in bed before rising.*
- *Attend to the natural urges of your colon when they arise.*

TRIPHALA

Triphala is an Ayurvedic herbal compound made up of three fruits or herbs – amalaki (*Embelica officinalis*), bibhitaki (*Terminalia belerica*), and haritaki (*Terminalia chebula*). The combination of the three herbs makes it a regulator of all three doshas. Triphala generally comes in powdered form, but many people prefer tablets or capsules because they do not like the taste.

Caution: *Do not take triphala in cases of diarrhoea or dysentery, or during pregnancy.*

Triphala has a laxative effect, but does not create dependency, nor disturb healthy intestinal flora. It regulates and rejuvenates the colon. It normalizes digestion and metabolism, and helps expel gases from the intestines. It aids weight reduction by assisting in the removal of toxins and fat from the cells. It is a source of vitamin C.

Triphala can be taken daily as a general tonic and bowel regulator. If you take it over a long period, then stop taking it for two to three weeks at approximately ten-week intervals. Although it is not addictive, the body will adapt to its regular long-term use, thereby making it less effective. It is best to take triphala in the evening, at least one and a half to two hours after food, and about half an hour before going to bed. In any case, do not eat for one and a half hours afterward.

You will need to find out how much triphala is right for you. Do not exceed 5 ml (one teaspoon) per day. When you start taking it, use a smaller amount, such as 1.25–2.5 ml (quarter or half of a teaspoon), increasing the amount gradually. When you first take it you may experience an increase in passing wind. The triphala is not creating these gases but helping expel old gases trapped in pockets in the intestines. If you experience loose stools when you start taking triphala, reduce the amount of triphala.

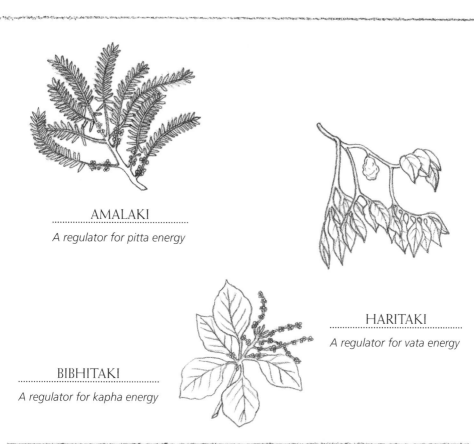

AMALAKI

A regulator for pitta energy

HARITAKI

A regulator for vata energy

BIBHITAKI

A regulator for kapha energy

Preparing Triphala
Triphala can be prepared in a number of ways. Try each of them to discover which suits you and your routine best. The strongest action will be obtained by simmering the triphala, and the weakest by soaking it and leaving the dregs.

- *Soak it in a cup of water at room temperature for eight hours. Drink the water, leaving the dregs.*
- *Mix it in a cup of tepid water and drink the water and the dregs.*
- *Put it in a cup and fill with boiling water. Leave to "brew" for 5 minutes before drinking. You can drink it either with or without the dregs.*
- *Simmer with about one and a half cups of water in a pan for 20 minutes – or longer if you want it stronger. Strain and drink.*

Food and Diet

मात्रावद्द्रव्यशनमशितमनुपहत्य प्रकृतिं
बलवर्णसुखायुषा योजयत्युपयोक्तारमवश्यमिति ॥

*Taken in appropriate quantity, food certainly helps the individual in bringing about
strength, complexion, happiness, and longevity without disturbing the equilibrium
of dhatus (tissues) and doshas of the body.*
(**Charaka Samhita** *Chapter 5: 8*)

For thousands of years, Ayurveda has taught that what
we eat plays a big part in determining health. All matter
consists of the five elements (see p. 22), which are a manifestation of consciousness. As you eat you take into yourself the subtle influences attached to the food and prana as
well as the physical form of the food. Even the stages of
production to which food is subjected affect its qualities.
Food is part of the dynamic dance of life and its qualities,
both obvious and subtle, affect your wellbeing.

The immediate connection between the qualities of
food and their impact on your health is not always obvious,
due in part to the complexities of Western diets and the
effects the digestive process has on food. *Charaka Samhita*
lists eight specific factors that you should take into account
when determining a diet appropriate for you. Consider
your diet in relation to these factors, since each will, to
some degree, help you determine if your diet is right for
you in your current circumstances, or indicate where you
could make beneficial changes.

The eight factors listed by *Charaka Samhita* are:
1. The natural qualities in foods
2. How the natural qualities in foods can be altered
3. The effects of combining foods
4. The quantity of food eaten
5. The place(s) and climate where the food was grown, prepared, and eaten
6. The effects of the seasons and time of day
7. General guidance on eating habits
8. Individual differences in the consumer of the food

Food Charts

Before looking at each of these factors, the following pages provide an overall classification of foods according to whether they tend to increase or pacify each dosha. Prepared by Dr. Vasant Lad, Director of the Ayurvedic Institute, Albuquerque, New Mexico, these charts take into account the combined effects of the tastes, energetics, and post-digestive effects of the foods (see Chapter Three) and their qualities (see p. 144). The charts are general and are designed to help everyone, so let your individual circumstances and tolerances guide you. Remember, too, that different methods of preparation and combination may modify the effects of the foods on your doshas.

You may find that, on first looking at these charts, your favourite foods are in the column that increase your predominant dosha (see Constitutional Assessment on pp. 38-41). This is understandable, since you are attracted to things that have similar qualities to yourself, as the principle "like attracts like" suggests.

One way to become familiar with this classification of foods is to copy the list, display it prominently (e.g. on the refrigerator door), and refer to it while you prepare meals. As you cook, look on the list to see the doshic classification of the foods you are using. If your meals are prepared for you, then daily review what you have eaten against the list.

When you start using Ayurvedic principles to adjust your diet, have a copy of the list with you when shopping. If you refer to it when selecting food, you will develop new shopping habits and be less likely to arrive home with items that are unsuitable for your doshic needs.

Assessing your Current Diet

Learning to classify your food – and hence your overall diet – as increasing or pacifying vata, pitta, or kapha, gives you the starting point for making changes. To do this, keep a record of everything you eat and drink for at least seven days. Remember to record all snacks and nibbles as well as meals, and the times when you ate them. For each day, use headings of breakfast, lunch, evening meal, and snacks. Leave space to note later whether the foods tend to increase or pacify vata, pitta, or kapha; and make notes, too, about how your food combinations affect your overall doshic picture and digestion (see Chapter Three).

You may find recording your diet a hard exercise. Not only do you have to remember to write it down, but if you snack frequently or eat foods judged as "bad", then seeing it written down may make you feel guilty. If you have a problem making your dietary record, regard it as an exercise in observation, and accept yourself as you are. Be kind and gentle with yourself. Guilt or shame may make you want to eat more, leading to more guilt and self-recrimination. Knowing what you are eating means that you are in a better position to make permanent changes, if that is what you choose.

With the qualities of the doshas (see Chapter Two) and the food charts to guide you, analyze your dietary record to see if foods that increase one dosha predominate in your diet. Use a different coloured pen for each dosha and mark the food items for each meal according to which dosha they increase.

Food Charts

The following pages give lists of foods that influence vata, pitta, and kapha. Each dosha contains two lists:
NO *means that the foods aggravate/increase the dosha. Avoid eating these foods if you are following a diet which pacifies the dosha.*
YES *means that the foods pacify/decrease the dosha. Select foods from this column if you are following a diet that pacifies the dosha.*

FOOD CHARTS

The Ayurvedic Institute

Food Guidelines for Basic Constitutional Types

NOTE: Guidelines provided in this table are general. Specific adjustments for individual requirements may need to be made, e.g. food allergies, strength of agni, season of the year, and degree of dosha predominance or aggravation.

* OK in moderation ‡ OK occasionally

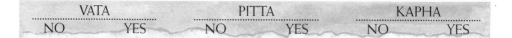

VATA		PITTA		KAPHA	
NO	YES	NO	YES	NO	YES

FRUITS

Generally most dried fruit	Generally most sweet fruit	Generally most sour fruit	Generally most sweet fruit	Generally most sweet & sour fruit	Generally most astringent fruit
Apples (raw)	Apples (cooked)	Apples (sour)	Apples (sweet)	Avocado	Apples
Cranberries	Apple sauce	Apricots (sour)	Apple sauce	Bananas	Apple sauce
Dates (dry)	Apricots	Bananas	Apricots	Coconut	Apricots
Figs (dry)	Avocado	Berries (sour)	(sweet)	Dates	Berries
Pears	Bananas	Cherries (sour)	Avocado	Figs (fresh)	Cherries
Persimmons	Berries	Cranberries	Berries (sweet)	Grapefruit	Cranberries
Pomegranates	Cherries	Grapefruit	Cherries	Grapes*	Figs (dry)*
Raisins (dry)	Coconut	Grapes (green)	(sweet)	Kiwi	Peaches
Prunes (dry)	Dates (fresh)	Kiwi‡	Coconut	Lemons*	Pears
Watermelon	Figs (fresh)	Lemons	Dates	Limes*	Persimmons
	Grapefruit	Mangoes	Figs	Mangoes‡	Pomegranates
	Grapes	(green)	Grapes (red &	Melons	Prunes
	Kiwi	Oranges (sour)	purple)	Oranges	Raisins
	Lemons	Papaya*	Limes*	Papaya	Strawberries*
	Limes	Peaches	Mangoes (ripe)	Pineapple	
	Mangoes	Persimmons	Melons	Plums	
	Melons	Pineapple	Oranges	Rhubarb	
	Oranges	(sour)	(sweet)	Tamarind	
	Papaya	Plums (sour)	Pears	Watermelon	
	Peaches	Rhubarb	Pineapple		
	Pineapple	Strawberries	(sweet)		
	Plums	Tamarind	Plums (sweet)		
	Prunes		Pomegranates		
	(soaked)		Prunes		
	Raisins		Raisins		
	(soaked)		Watermelon		
	Rhubarb				
	Strawberries				
	Tamarind				

VATA		PITTA		KAPHA	
NO	YES	NO	YES	NO	YES

DAIRY

NO	YES	NO	YES	NO	YES
Cheese (hard)*	Most dairy is good!	Butter (salted)	Butter (unsalted)	Butter (salted)	Butter (unsalted)‡
Cow's milk (powdered)	Butter	Buttermilk	Cheese (soft, not aged, unsalted)	Buttermilk*	Cottage cheese (from skimmed goat's milk)
Goat's milk (powdered)	Buttermilk	Cheese (hard)	Cottage cheese	Cheese (soft & hard)	
Yogurt (plain, frozen or w/th fruit)	Cheese (soft)	Sour cream	Cow's milk	Cow's milk	Ghee*
	Cottage cheese	Yogurt (plain, frozen or w/th fruit)	Ghee	Ice cream	Goat's cheese (unsalted & not aged)*
	Cow's milk		Goat's milk	Sour cream	
	Ghee		Goat's cheese (soft, unsalted)	Yogurt (plain, frozen or with fruit)	Ghee*
	Goat's cheese		Ice cream		Goat's milk (skimmed only)
	Goat's milk		Yogurt (freshly made & diluted)		Yogurt (diluted)
	Ice cream*				
	Sour cream*				
	Yogurt (diluted & spiced)*				

VEGETABLES

NO	YES	NO	YES	NO	YES
Generally frozen, raw, or dried vegetables	In general vegetables should be cooked	In general pungent vegetables	In general sweet & bitter vegetables	In general sweet & juicy vegetables	In general most pungent & bitter vegetables
Artichoke	Asparagus	Beet greens	Artichoke	Cucumber	Artichoke
Beet greens‡	Beets	Beets (raw)	Asparagus	Olives, black or green‡	Asparagus
Bitter melon	Cabbage*	Burdock root	Beets (cooked)	Parsnips‡	Beet greens
Broccoli	Carrots	Carrots (raw)*	Bitter melon	Potatoes, sweet	Beets
Brussels sprouts	Cauliflower*	Corn (fresh)‡	Broccoli	Pumpkin	Bitter melon
Burdock root	Cilantro	Daikon radish	Brussels sprouts	Spaghetti squash*	Broccoli
Cabbage (raw)	Cucumber	Eggplant‡	Cabbage	Squash, winter	Brussels sprouts
Cauliflower (raw)	Daikon radish*	Garlic	Carrots (cooked)	Taro root	Burdock root
Celery	Fennel (Anise)	Green chillies	Cauliflower	Tomatoes (raw)	Cabbage
Corn (fresh)‡	Garlic	Horseradish	Celery	Zucchini	Carrots
Dandelion greens	Green beans	Kohlrabi‡	Cilantro		Cauliflower
Eggplant	Green chillies	Leeks (raw)	Cucumber		Celery
Jerusalem artichoke*	Horseradish‡	Mustard greens	Dandelion greens		Cilantro
Kale	Leeks	Olives, green	Fennel (Anise)		Corn
Kohlrabi	Mustard greens*	Onions (raw)	Green beans		Daikon radish
Leafy greens*	Okra	Peppers (hot)	Jerusalem artichoke		Dandelion greens
Lettuce*	Olives, black	Prickly pear (fruit)	Kale		Eggplant
Mushrooms	Onions (cooked)*	Radishes (raw)	Leafy greens		Fennel (Anise)
Olives, green	Parsnip	Spinach (raw)	Leeks (cooked)		Garlic
Onions (raw)	Peas (cooked)	Tomatoes	Lettuce		Green beans
Parsley*	Potatoes, sweet	Turnip greens	Mushrooms		Green chillies
Peas (raw)	Pumpkin	Turnips	Okra		Horseradish
Peppers, sweet & hot	Radishes (cooked)*		Olives, black		Jerusalem artichoke
			Onions (cooked)		

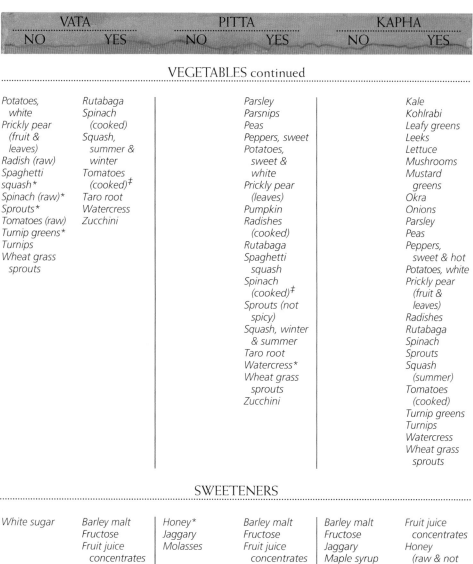

VATA		PITTA		KAPHA	
NO	YES	NO	YES	NO	YES

VEGETABLES continued

Potatoes, white	Rutabaga		Parsley		Kale
Prickly pear (fruit & leaves)	Spinach (cooked)		Parsnips		Kohlrabi
	Squash, summer & winter		Peas		Leafy greens
Radish (raw)	Tomatoes (cooked)‡		Peppers, sweet		Leeks
Spaghetti squash*	Taro root		Potatoes, sweet & white		Lettuce
Spinach (raw)*	Watercress		Prickly pear (leaves)		Mushrooms
Sprouts*	Zucchini		Pumpkin		Mustard greens
Tomatoes (raw)			Radishes (cooked)		Okra
Turnip greens*			Rutabaga		Onions
Turnips			Spaghetti squash		Parsley
Wheat grass sprouts			Spinach (cooked)‡		Peas
			Sprouts (not spicy)		Peppers, sweet & hot
			Squash, winter & summer		Potatoes, white
			Taro root		Prickly pear (fruit & leaves)
			Watercress*		Radishes
			Wheat grass sprouts		Rutabaga
			Zucchini		Spinach
					Sprouts
					Squash (summer)
					Tomatoes (cooked)
					Turnip greens
					Turnips
					Watercress
					Wheat grass sprouts

SWEETENERS

White sugar	Barley malt	Honey*	Barley malt	Barley malt	Fruit juice concentrates
	Fructose	Jaggary	Fructose	Fructose	Honey (raw & not processed)
	Fruit juice concentrates	Molasses	Fruit juice concentrates	Jaggary	
	Honey		Maple syrup	Maple syrup	
	Jaggary		Rice syrup	Molasses	
	Maple syrup‡		Sucanat	Rice syrup	
	Molasses		Turbinado	Sucanat	
	Rice syrup		White sugar‡	Turbinado	
	Sucanat			White sugar	
	Turbinado				

VATA		PITTA		KAPHA	
NO	YES	NO	YES	NO	YES

LEGUMES

Aduki beans	Lentils (red)*	Miso	Aduki beans	Kidney beans	Aduki beans
Black beans	Miso‡	Soy sauce	Black beans	Mung beans*	Black beans
Black-eyed	Mung beans	Soy sausages	Black-eyed peas	Mung dal*	Black-eyed
peas	Mung dal	Tur dal	Chick peas	Soy beans	peas
Chick peas	Soy cheese*	Urad dal	(Garbanzos)	Soy cheese	Chick Peas
(Garbanzos)	Soy milk*		Kidney beans	Soy flour	(Garbanzos)
Kidney beans	Soy sauce*		Lentils (brown	Soy powder	Lentils (red &
Lentils (brown)	Soy sausages*		& red)	Soy sauce	brown)
Lima beans	Tur dal		Lima beans	Tofu (cold)	Lima beans
Navy beans	Urad dal		Mung beans	Urad dal	Miso
Peas (dried)			Mung dal		Navy beans
Pinto beans			Navy beans		Peas (dried)
Soy beans			Peas (dried)		Pinto beans
Soy flour			Pinto beans		Soy milk
Soy powder			Soy beans		Soy sausages
Split peas			Soy cheese		Split peas
Tempeh			Soy flour*		Tempeh
Tofu*			Soy milk		Tofu (hot)*
White beans			Soy powder*		Tur dal
			Split peas		White beans
			Tempeh		
			Tofu		
			White beans		

ANIMAL FOODS

Chicken	Beef	Beef	Buffalo	Beef	Chicken
(white)*	Buffalo	Chicken (dark)	Chicken	Buffalo	(white)
Lamb	Chicken (dark)	Duck	(white)	Chicken (dark)	Eggs
Pork	Duck	Eggs (yolk)	Eggs (albumen	Duck	Fish (freshwater)
Rabbit	Eggs	Fish (sea)	or white	Fish (sea)	Rabbit
Venison	Fish (freshwater	Lamb	only)	Lamb	Shrimp
Turkey (white)	or sea)	Pork	Fish (freshwater)	Pork	Turkey (white)
	Salmon	Salmon	Rabbit	Salmon	Venison
	Sardines	Sardines	Shrimp*	Sardines	
	Seafood	Seafood	Turkey (white)	Seafood	
	Shrimp	Tuna fish	Venison	Tuna fish	
	Tuna fish	Turkey (dark)		Turkey (dark)	
	Turkey (dark)				

VATA		PITTA		KAPHA	
NO	YES	NO	YES	NO	YES

CONDIMENTS

Chilli peppers*	Black pepper*	Chocolate	Black pepper*	Chocolate	Black pepper
Chocolate	Chutney,	Chutney,	Chutney,	Chutney,	Chilli peppers
Horseradish	mango (sweet	mango	mango	mango	Chutney,
Sprouts*	or spicy)	(spicy)	(sweet)	(sweet)	mango
	Coriander	Dulse*	Coriander	Dulse*	(spicy)
	leaves*	Gomasio	leaves	Gomasio	Coriander
	Dulse	Horseradish	Hijiki*	Hijiki*	leaves
	Gomasio	Kelp	Kombu*	Kelp	Horseradish
	Hijiki	Ketchup	Lime*	Ketchup‡	Mustard
	Kelp	Mustard	Sprouts	Lemon*	(without
	Ketchup	Lemon		Lime	vinegar)
	Kombu	Lime pickle		Lime pickle	Scallions
	Lemon	Mango pickle		Mango pickle	Sprouts
	Lime	Mayonnaise		Mayonnaise	
	Lime pickle	Pickles		Pickles	
	Mango pickle	Salt (in excess)		Salt	
	Mayonnaise	Scallions		Seaweed*	
	Mustard	Seaweed		Soy sauce	
	Pickles	Soy sauce		Tamari	
	Salt	Tamari*		Vinegar	
	Scallions	Vinegar			
	Seaweed				
	Soy sauce				
	Tamari				
	Vinegar				
	Chilli peppers				

NUTS

None	In moderation:	Almonds	Almonds	Almonds	Charole
	Almonds	(with skin)	(soaked and	(soaked &	
	Black walnuts	Black walnuts	peeled)	peeled)‡	
	Brazil nuts	Brazil nuts	Charole	Black walnuts	
	Cashews	Cashews	Coconut	Brazil nuts	
	Charole	Filberts		Cashews	
	Coconut	Hazelnuts		Coconut	
	Filberts	Macadamia		Filberts	
	Hazelnuts	nuts		Hazelnuts	
	Macadamia	Peanuts		Macadamia	
	nuts	Pecans		nuts	
	Peanuts‡	Pine nuts		Peanuts	
	Pecans	Pistachios		Pecans	
	Pine nuts	Walnuts		Pine nuts	
	Pistachios			Pistachios	
	Walnuts			Walnuts	

VATA		PITTA		KAPHA	
NO	YES	NO	YES	NO	YES

BEVERAGES

VATA NO	VATA YES	PITTA NO	PITTA YES	KAPHA NO	KAPHA YES
Apple juice	Alcohol (beer	Alcohol (spirits	Alcohol, beer*	Alcohol (beer,	Alcohol
Black tea	or wine)*	or wine)	Almond milk	spirits, sweet	(dry wine, red
Caffeinated	Almond milk	Apple cider	Aloe vera juice	wine)	or white)
beverages	Aloe vera juice	Berry juice	Apple juice	Almond milk	Aloe vera juice
Carbonated	Apple cider	(sour)	Apricot juice	Caffeinated	Apple cider
drinks	Apricot juice	Caffeinated	Berry juice	beverages‡	Apple juice*
Carob*	Berry juice	beverages	(sweet)	Carbonated	Apricot juice
Chocolate milk	(except	Carbonated	Black tea	drinks	Berry juice
Coffee	cranberry)	drinks	Carob	Chai (hot,	Black tea
Cold dairy	Carrot juice	Carrot juice	Chai (hot,	spiced milk)*	(spiced)
drinks	Chai (hot	Cherry juice	spiced milk)*	Cherry juice	Carob
Cranberry juice	spiced milk)	(sour)	Cherry juice	(sour)	Carrot juice
Iced tea	Cherry juice	Chocolate milk	(sweet)	Chocolate milk	Cherry juice
Icy cold drinks	Grain 'coffee'	Coffee	Cool dairy	Coffee	(sweet)
Mixed veg.	Grape juice	Cranberry juice	drinks	Cold dairy	Cranberry juice
juice	Grapefruit	Grapefruit	Grain 'coffee'	drinks	Grain 'coffee'
Pear juice	juice	juice	Grape juice	Grapefruit	Grape juice
Pomegranate	Lemonade	Iced tea	Mango juice	juice	Mango juice
juice	Mango juice	Icy cold drinks	Mixed veg. juice	Iced tea	Mixed veg. juice
Prune juice‡	Miso broth	Lemonade	Peach nectar	Icy cold drinks	Peach nectar
Soy milk (cold)	Orange juice	Orange juice*	Pear juice	Lemonade	Pear juice
Tomato juice‡	Papaya juice	Miso broth*	Pomegranate	Miso broth	Pomegranate
V-8 Juice	Peach nectar	Papaya juice	juice	Orange juice	juice
Vegetable	Pineapple juice	Pineapple juice	Prune juice	Papaya juice	Prune juice
bouillon	Rice milk	Tomato juice	Rice milk	Pineapple	Soy milk (hot &
	Sour juices	V-8 juice	Soy milk	juice*	well-spiced)
Herb teas:	Soy milk (hot &	Sour juices	Vegetable	Rice milk	Vegetable
Alfalfa‡	well-spiced)*		bouillon	Sour juices	bouillon
Barley‡		**Herb teas:**		Soy milk (cold)	
Blackberry	**Herb teas:**	Ajwan	**Herb teas:**	Tomato juice	**Herb teas:**
Borage‡	Ajwan	Basil‡	Alfalfa	V-8 Juice	Ajwan
Burdock	Bancha	Cinnamon‡	Bancha		Alfalfa
Catnip*	Basil‡	Clove	Barley	**Herb teas:**	Barley
Chicory*	Chamomile	Eucalyptus	Blackberry	Comfrey*	Basil
Chrysanthemum*	Cinnamon‡	Fenugreek	Borage	Marshmallow	Blackberry
Cornsilk	Clove	Ginger (dry)	Burdock	Red zinger	Borage
Dandelion	Comfrey	Ginseng	Catnip	Rosehip‡	Burdock
Ginseng	Elderflower	Hawthorn	Chamomile		Catnip
Hibiscus	Eucalyptus	Hyssop	Chicory		Chamomile
Hops‡	Fennel	Juniper berry	Chrysanthemum		Chicory
Hyssop‡	Fenugreek	Mormon tea	Comfrey		Chrysanthemum
Jasmine‡	Ginger (fresh)	Pennyroyal	Cornsilk		Cinnamon
Lemon balm‡	Hawthorn	Red zinger	Dandelion		Clove
Mormon tea	Juniper berry	Rosehip‡	Elderflower		Corn silk
Nettle‡	Kukicha*	Sage	Fennel		Dandelion
Passion	Lavender	Sassafras	Ginger (fresh)		Elder flower
flower‡	Lemon grass	Yerba mate	Hibiscus		Eucalyptus
Red clover‡	Licorice		Hops		Fennel*
Red zinger‡	Marshmallow		Jasmine		Fenugreek

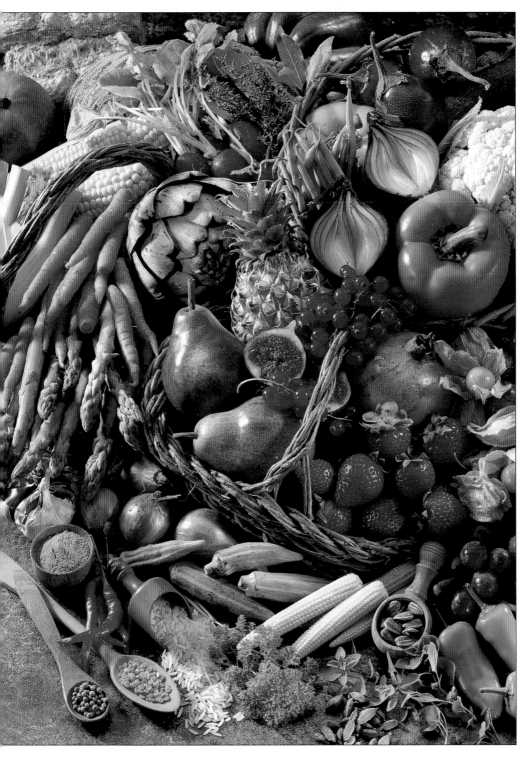

All the foods you eat have qualities which influence your doshas.

VATA		PITTA		KAPHA	
NO	YES	NO	YES	NO	YES

BEVERAGES continued

VATA		PITTA		KAPHA	
NO	YES	NO	YES	NO	YES
Sage	Oat straw		Kukicha		Ginger
Strawberry*	Orange peel		Lavender		Ginseng*
Violet‡	Pennyroyal		Lemon balm		Hibiscus
Wintergreen*	Peppermint		Lemon grass		Hops
Yarrow	Raspberry*		Licorice		Hyssop
Yerba mate‡	Rosehip		Marshmallow		Jasmine
	Saffron		Nettle		Juniper berry
	Sarsaparilla		Oat straw		Kukicha
	Sassafras		Orange peel*		Lavender
	Spearmint		Passion flower		Lemon balm
			Peppermint		Lemon grass
			Raspberry		Licorice*
			Red clover		Mormon tea
			Saffron		Nettle
			Sarsaparilla		Oat straw
			Spearmint		Orange peel
			Strawberry		Passion flower
			Violet		Pennyroyal
			Wintergreen		Peppermint
			Yarrow		Raspberry
					Red clover
					Saffron
					Sage
					Sarsaparilla*
					Sassafras
					Spearmint
					Strawberry
					Violet
					Wintergreen
					Yarrow
					Yerba mate

SEEDS

VATA		PITTA		KAPHA	
NO	YES	NO	YES	NO	YES
Popcorn	Chia	Chia	Flax	Halva	Chia
	Flax	Sesame	Halva	Sesame	Flax*
	Halva	Tahini	Popcorn (no	Tahini	Popcorn (no
	Psyllium‡		salt,		salt, no
	Pumpkin		buttered)		butter)
	Sesame		Psyllium		Psyllium‡
	Sunflower		Pumpkin*		Pumpkin*
	Tahini		Sunflower		Sunflower*

VATA		PITTA		KAPHA	
NO	YES	NO	YES	NO	YES

SPICES

Caraway	All spices are good! Ajwan Allspice Almond extract Anise Asafoetida (hing) Basil Bay leaf Black pepper Cardamon Cayenne* Cinnamon Cloves Coriander Cumin Dill Fennel Fenugreek* Garlic Ginger Mace Marjoram Mint Mustard seeds Neem leaves Nutmeg Orange peel Oregano Paprika Parsley Peppermint Pippali Poppy seeds Rosemary Saffron Sage Salt Savory Spearmint Star anise Tarragon Thyme Turmeric Vanilla Wintergreen	Ajwan Allspice Almond extract Anise Asafoetida (hing) Basil (dry) Bay leaf Caraway* Cayenne Cloves Fenugreek Garlic Ginger (dry) Mace Marjoram Mustard seeds Nutmeg Oregano Paprika Pippali Poppy seeds Rosemary Sage Salt Savory Star anise Tarragon* Thyme	Basil (fresh) Black pepper* Cardamon* Cinnamon Coriander Cumin Dill Fennel Ginger (fresh) Mint Neem leaves* Orange peel* Parsley* Peppermint Saffron Spearmint Turmeric Vanilla* Wintergreen	Salt	All spices are good! Ajwan Allspice Almond extract Anise Asafoetida (hing) Basil Bay leaf Black pepper Caraway Cardamon Cayenne Cinnamon Cloves Coriander Cumin Dill Fennel* Fenugreek Garlic Ginger Mace Marjoram Mint Mustard seeds Neem leaves Nutmeg Orange peel Oregano Paprika Parsley Peppermint Pippali Poppy seeds Rosemary Saffron Sage Savory Spearmint Star anise Tarragon Thyme Turmeric Vanilla* Wintergreen

VATA		PITTA		KAPHA	
NO	YES	NO	YES	NO	YES

GRAINS§

VATA NO	VATA YES	PITTA NO	PITTA YES	KAPHA NO	KAPHA YES
Barley	Amaranth*	Bread (with	Amaranth	Bread (with	Amaranth*
Bread (with	Durham flour	yeast)	Barley	yeast)	Barley
yeast)	Oats (cooked)	Buckwheat	Cereal, dry	Oats (cooked)	Buckwheat
Buckwheat	Pancakes	Corn	Couscous	Pancakes	Cereal (cold,
Cereals (cold,	Quinoa	Millet	Crackers	Pasta‡	dry, or
dry, or	Rice (all kinds)	Muesli‡	Durham flour	Quinoa*	puffed)
puffed)	Seitan (wheat	Oats (dry)	Granola	Rice (brown,	Corn
Corn	meat)	Polenta‡	Oat bran	white)	Couscous
Couscous	Sprouted	Quinoa	Oats (cooked)	Rice cakes‡	Crackers
Crackers	wheat bread	Rice (brown)‡	Pancakes	Spelt*	Durham flour*
Granola	(Essene)	Rye	Pasta	Wheat	Granola
Millet	Wheat		Rice (basmati,		Millet
Muesli			white, wild)		Muesli
Oat bran			Rice cakes		Oat bran
Oats (dry)			Sago		Oats (dry)
Pasta‡			Seitan (wheat		Polenta
Polenta‡			meat)		Rice (basmati,
Rice cakes‡			Spelt		wild)*
Rye			Sprouted		Rye
Sago			wheat bread		Sago
Spelt			(Essene)		Seitan (wheat
Tapioca			Tapioca		meat)
Wheat bran			Wheat		Sprouted
			Wheat bran		wheat bread
					(Essene)
					Tapioca
					Wheat bran

§Always use suitable grains when 'generic' things are listed

OILS

VATA NO	VATA YES	PITTA NO	PITTA YES	KAPHA NO	KAPHA YES
Flax seed	For internal &	Almond	For internal &	Avocado	For internal &
	external use	Apricot	external use	Apricot	external use in
	(most suitable	Corn	(most suitable	Coconut	small amounts
	at top of list):	Safflower	at top of list):	Olive	(most suitable
	Sesame	Sesame	Sunflower	Primrose	at top of list):
	Ghee		Ghee	Safflower	Corn
	Olive		Canola	Sesame	Canola
	Most other oils		Olive	Soy	Sunflower
			Soy	Walnut	Ghee
	External use		Flax seed		Almond
	only:		Primrose		Flax seed‡
	Coconut		Walnut		
	Avocado				
			External use		
			only:		
			Avocado		
			Coconut		

VATA		PITTA		KAPHA	
NO	YES	NO	YES	NO	YES

FOOD SUPPLEMENTS

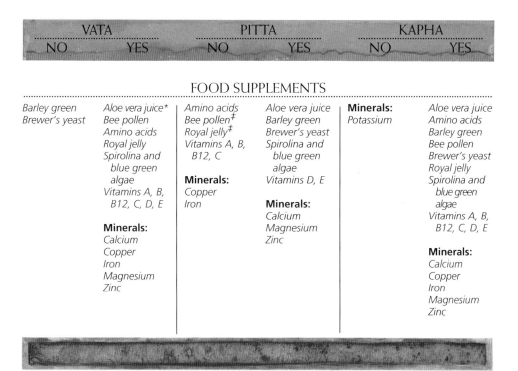

Barley green	Aloe vera juice*	Amino acids	Aloe vera juice	**Minerals:**	Aloe vera juice
Brewer's yeast	Bee pollen	Bee pollen‡	Barley green	Potassium	Amino acids
	Amino acids	Royal jelly‡	Brewer's yeast		Barley green
	Royal jelly	Vitamins A, B,	Spirolina and		Bee pollen
	Spirolina and	B12, C	blue green		Brewer's yeast
	blue green		algae		Royal jelly
	algae	**Minerals:**	Vitamins D, E		Spirolina and
	Vitamins A, B,	Copper			blue green
	B12, C, D, E	Iron	**Minerals:**		algae
			Calcium		Vitamins A, B,
	Minerals:		Magnesium		B12, C, D, E
	Calcium		Zinc		
	Copper				**Minerals:**
	Iron				Calcium
	Magnesium				Copper
	Zinc				Iron
					Magnesium
					Zinc

A Word of Caution:

These are guidelines only, and not meant to substitute in any way for the advice of a qualified physician or nutritionist. Ayurveda always recommends a slow and steady approach to changes in your diet. Do not try to do everything at once!

After you have discovered which diet is for you (see pp. 154-5), remember to listen closely to your body as you try different foods. If for instance you get gas, or heartburn, it may not be the food for you. Everyone is completely individual, and even though the food is on your list, it might not agree with you. So be gentle and loving with yourself. Slowly with this list and your own listening will come a way of eating that will bring great balance and health into your life. Also Ayurveda says that it is not what you eat occasionally that creates a serious imbalance, but what you consume on a day-by-day basis.

The Natural Qualities of Food

All foods have obvious and subtle qualities which affect your physical body and influence your doshas. Three contrasting pairs of natural qualities (see p. 32) which are most useful when first considering the effects of these qualities are: light–heavy; liquid/oily–drying; heating/hot–cooling/cold (the latter refers to both temperature and energetics – see pp. 52-3).

Select foods which have the natural qualities to give the results you desire. For instance, if your body is dry (signs include dry skin or hard dry stools), avoid drying foods and tastes (see pp. 54-5). You can change the qualities of food – for example, by steaming vegetables rather than eating them raw, or by adding an oil dressing. If there is too much heat in your body (one indication might be an itchy rash), cut down on "hot" foods, i.e. those that increase pitta.

Raw foods are often advocated to add roughage to the diet and if you suffer from constipation you may notice an initial improvement. But, in the long term, the roughness of too much raw food may increase vata and so contribute to the constipation.

Foods and their Qualities
The table gives examples of qualities of some of the foods we eat. We may only become aware of the effects of qualities in foods after we have been eating them regularly for some time. Even then we may not always relate the changes in our bodies to those foods.

NATURAL QUALITIES

Heavy	Milk~Wheat~Brown rice~Fish~Red meat~Sesame oil
Light	Mung beans~Basmati rice~Leafy vegetables Chicken~Apple~Sunflower oil
Cooling/Cold	Milk~Sunflower oil~Wheat~Apple~Ice cream~Coconut
Heating/Hot	Fish~Sesame oil~Onions~Eggs~Meat~Chilli
Oily	Most nuts~Fish~Eggs
Drying	Many vegetables~Pears~Millet

ALTERING FOOD'S NATURAL QUALITIES

The natural qualities of foods can be changed in obvious
ways, such as cooking, but also in subtle ways – for example, through the attitudes of those involved in growing,
preparing, and marketing food.

Cooking alters the qualities of food. Cold foods can be
made hot; dry foods made moist or oily. For instance, the
qualities of muesli with cold milk are dry, cold, and heavy –
qualities which increase vata and kapha. Oats made into
porridge are a more suitable breakfast if you are following a
vata-pacifying diet, because you have imparted moisture
and warmth to the oats.

Although foods do not have a prana rating, lack of prana
in your food will lead to low vitality and eventually fatigue
(see pp. 50-1). Modern methods of production, processing,
packaging, and distribution reduce the prana in food and
microwave cooking may destroy it. Some processed foods
contain substances to please the senses. Such substances,
rather than adding nutrients that the body can use for
healthy tissue building, may distort the body's natural intelligence and lead to ama. They may even make the mind
crave inappropriate foods.

Ayurveda teaches that subtle influences can affect us,
and so the attitudes and emotions of those who prepare
food will be imparted to it, so it is best to eat food cooked
with love. Food cooked in anger may subtly upset the
digestion. The subtle qualities of many processed foods are
not known nor are all the long-term effects of their habitual use. Any food taken in inappropriate circumstances or in
excess will be "bad". What is inappropriate or excessive will
vary for each person and their current doshic balance. Even
"healthy" foods can be misused and create ama: raw honey
in small quantities is beneficial, but cooked honey cannot
be assimilated and will create ama. We cannot always
escape these influences, but we should be aware of them so
that we can select, as far as possible, fresh foods that have
been subjected to a minimum of commercial processing.

Bad Influences

It is likely that some manu-
factured products, which
are designed to replace
foods currently considered
"bad" for you (such as sugar
and butter), may not be
made into healthy tissues;
and if they are not expelled
from the body they will
result in ama and blocked
channels.

COMBINING FOODS

According to the teachings in Ayurveda, particular foods should not be combined because they put a strain on the digestive process. All substances have their own tastes, energetics, and post-digestive effects (see pp. 52-3), which influence how the food is digested and utilized. The different digestive demands of foods eaten at the same meal may strain the digestive system and deplete agni. Such foods, when eaten at separate meals, may, however, be properly digested and so add to your wellbeing.

The antagonistic qualities of foods that are not ideally combined may be reduced by one-pot cooking (see right).

Unfortunately, the rules about food combining cannot be simply set out as a comprehensive table that says "Do not eat this with that". As with all things in Ayurveda, everything is relative and general rules have to be applied individually. If your digestion is poor you need to take more care about combining foods than if you have a strong digestive capacity.

It is essential that you learn to understand not only what your body is telling you but also the state of your agni or digestive capabilities, which will vary from time to time. You may already know that some foods do not agree with you, or that sometimes they do and on other occasions they do not. Your own observation is a good teacher.

One-pot Cooking

If you cook together foods of different tastes, energetics, or post-digestive effects (see pp. 52-3) in one pot, such as a casserole, you can substantially reduce the adverse effects of incompatible food combinations. The foods are formed into one "juice" that acts upon the digestive system. One-pot cooking is a good way to help settle the irregularities of excess vata on digestion (see p. 162 for the recipe for kitcheri).

Some General Rules about Food Combining
- Do not mix foods that have different energetic characteristics (see pp. 52-3) at the same meal. For example, do not mix milk, which is cooling, with fish or meat, which are both heating.
- Do not eat cooked and raw foods at the same meal. Raw foods are harder to digest.
- Do not eat fruit with other foods.
- Do not mix milk and yogurt.
- Do not mix milk or yogurt with sour or citrus fruits, fish, meat, eggs, nightshades (potatoes, tomatoes, or aubergine), or starches.
- Do not mix different types of protein, such as eggs and cheese.

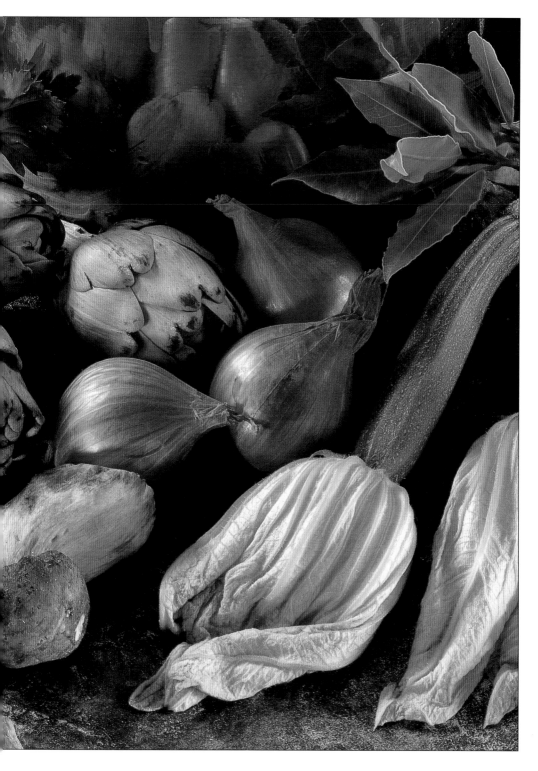

Quantity of Food

How much food you eat should primarily be related to your ability to digest it. You should eat neither too much nor too little. Think of the digestion process as a fire. A fire reduced to embers will go out if you add a large amount of fuel. But a few, light kindling sticks will ignite, increasing the fire and allowing further fuel to be burnt. Likewise a fire that receives too little fuel will go out. Always aim to eat the amount that will restore or maintain a steady digestion.

Your digestive capacity is related to your constitution. Vata types tend to undereat or eat erratically, which makes digestion irregular; kaphas tend to overeat, which slows down digestion. Pitta types are more likely to have good digestive strength, though too much hot spicy food will make their digestive fire burn too fiercely (see pp. 76-7).

Other factors that determine the right quantity to eat include age, level of activity, occupation, the season, and time of day. If you are under-eating or over-eating, do not suddenly change the quantity of food you eat, but regularly eat a little more or less over a period of weeks.

The advice in Ayurvedic texts about the optimum amount to eat at one meal varies between one third to one half of the stomach's capacity of solids, one quarter to one third for fluids, leaving one quarter to one third empty. Discover what suits you. In general, vata types should drink more fluids than kaphas. Fluids help in the digestion and absorption of the food; space is needed for the proper mixing with the digestive juices. Generally, when you are ill, you should eat a little less than you are hungry for.

It is vital to eat the right amount of individual foods. According to Ayurveda, a suitable diet is 40%-60% grains, 10%-20% protein, and 30%-50% vegetables and fruit. Adjust this according to your constitution. Kaphas could benefit by eating at least 40% of their diet as vegetables, because they are generally light, whereas vatas should have more grains than vegetables. About 10% of the diet for all doshas should be fruit, but not eaten with other foods.

Eating Meat

Ayurveda does not recommend meat as a regular part of the diet because it is heavy to digest. However, it can be eaten when necessary to strengthen the body, prepared in a way that assists its digestion, such as in soups or casseroles.

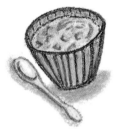

THE IMPORTANCE OF PLACE

The quality of, and the qualities in, food are influenced by the place where the food is grown and produced. Try to obtain food that has come from a wholesome environment – for example, from a non-polluted place with fertile soil, and grown by people who enjoy producing food.

When *Charaka Samhita* was written about 3000 years ago, most food would have been grown and prepared within the community that ate it. Nowadays, we need to consider the effects of foods brought in from other parts of the world as well as the effects on the subtle energies in food caused by modern methods of food production. The conditions in which animals live and die have a subtle influence on the products we consume from their carcasses. We may also ingest with our food residues of chemicals used in current agricultural methods. The subtle qualities of food grown in a naturally rich soil will differ from the qualities of food grown in a depleted soil with the aid of chemicals. The subtle energies of such chemicals may impair the normal functions of the doshas as well as creating ama.

The climate of your local environment should guide your decision when selecting foods. For example, if you live in an arid climate, foods with rough or sharp qualities will be antagonistic to your body. So, too, would cold, heavy foods eaten in a cold, damp place.

Climate and geographical locations are interlinked and have doshic qualities. Places at sea level and places with cold, wet climates have strong kapha qualities. Places at altitude and places with a low rainfall or a lot of wind have strong vata qualities. Sunshine brings pitta qualities. The ideal climate is a place such as Hawaii, where no doshic quality is excessive. If you move to a different environment your body will need time to adapt, and you may need to take extra measures to compensate. For example, moving to the altitude and dryness of New Mexico after a life by the ocean in California may increase your vata. If so, you should adapt your diet and oil your skin more often.

The Ideal Climate
The tropical islands of Hawaii are blessed with a balanced climate in which neither vata, pitta, nor kapha are excessive.

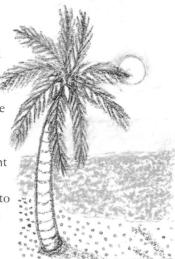

THE SEASONS OF THE YEAR

The natural progress through the stages of life (see p. 10), the changes in the seasons, and time of day are external factors over which you have no control. They all have qualities that can affect your health. If you understand these qualities then you are in a position to reduce possible adverse effects by incorporating the opposite qualities into your lifestyle. To some extent you already do this when you wear a warm coat in winter, or a sun hat in summer. By understanding the cycles of these external factors in relation to the qualities of VPK, you are in a better position to plan your lifestyle and diet to match your doshic needs (see also p. 61).

Adjust your diet to your stage of life, especially in the vata-age (55 and over) when you should eat raw and dry foods only occasionally. Also adjust your diet according to the seasons because of their effect on the doshas. In winter, you eat warmer and heavier foods than in summer, unless a constitutional or doshic imbalance indicates the contrary. In general, salads are more appropriate in the summer to cool pitta; ginger tea in winter to warm vata and kapha.

VPK and the Seasons
A dosha is naturally increased during the season that has similar qualities. You should take these seasonal changes into account in your eating habits and especially during the season which aggravates your predominant dosha.

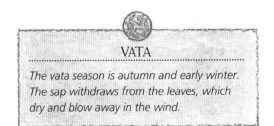

VATA

The vata season is autumn and early winter. The sap withdraws from the leaves, which dry and blow away in the wind.

PITTA

Pitta energy increases in late spring with the increase in temperature and throughout summer, the hottest part of the year and the longer sunny days.

KAPHA

The coldest part of winter when nature is frozen and solid is the season when kapha is naturally disturbed. The liquid quality of kapha is experienced during early spring with the melting of winter's ice, and the rising of the sap.

TIME OF DAY

The time you eat your meals also affects the doshic qualities of the meals. It is advisable not to eat late at night, and
to leave at least two hours before going to bed to allow for
digestion. If you have a kapha constitution or are following
a kapha-pacifying diet, remember that eating at kapha
times of the day will increase the heaviness of eating.
Breakfast is not generally recommended for those with a
kapha constitution for the same reason, but always take
your individual circumstances into account. If you are following a kapha-pacifying diet, eat breakfast before 7 am
and do not have your evening meal after 7 pm.

People with pitta constitutions should aim to have their
main meal around midday when the sun, pitta, and agni are
at their highest. If you have excess pitta you may be more
critical until you eat.

The main vata time is early morning. Late afternoon and
early evening are also vata times, the "autumn" of the day. If
you are dealing with excess vata or managing a vata constitution then the most important thing is to eat at regular
times. Breakfast around 8 am, lunch at 12.30 pm, and an
evening meal around 6 pm is probably the best for you.
Sometimes, however, you may need to eat smaller meals
four or even five times a day.

Daily Rhythms
*The rhythms of the day
have their own qualities of
VPK. The beginning of the
day, when movement and
activity begin, is the main
vata time. The middle part
of the day is the main pitta
time. Slowing down and
sleep come at the end of
the day, the principal kapha
time. Each of the three
doshas' energies peak to a
lesser extent at other times.
For example, the other pitta
time is midnight. An
ailment whose symptoms
are worse at midday or midnight is likely to be the
result of excess pitta.*

Main

Secondary

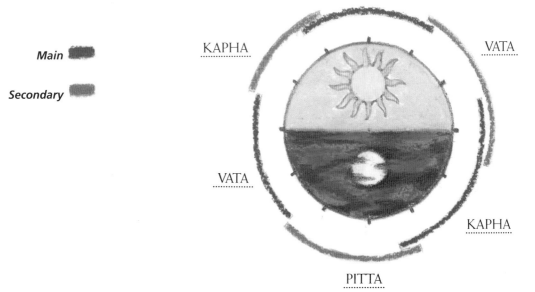

GENERAL RULES ABOUT DIET

The principles outlined on the preceding pages of this chapter will help guide you toward eating the appropriate amount, at appropriate times, of the right kinds of foods that do not disturb your doshas or agni. You are aiming to eat foods that: are compatible and easily digested, absorbed, and assimilated; provide your body's requirements for building tissues; and satisfy your senses and mind.

All the guidelines for choosing foods need adjustment to suit individual doshic requirements. However, some rules for good eating apply to almost everyone – and most of them are common sense.

- Is your desire to eat coming from your mind or body? Eat only when your body is naturally hungry.
- Do not eat until your stomach has finished working on the previous meal.
- Do not eat when you are very emotional, angry, worried, or upset, as this disturbs agni.
- Avoid incompatible food combinations.
- Do not over-eat or under-eat.
- Eat wholesome foods that are pleasing to the senses.
- Avoid foods you don't like, as they won't satisfy the mind.
- Avoid under-cooked, over-cooked, or burnt foods.
- Do not eat unripe or over-ripe fruits.
- Avoid eating leftovers, or habitually eating reheated foods, as they will have little prana.
- Do not drink iced water before, during, or immediately after a meal. Coldness shocks the body; it also inhibits agni and causes ama. If you wish to drink with your meals, have drinks that are warm, or a small amount of wine, which can aid digestion.
- Eat in congenial company or pleasant silence.
- When eating, do not talk too much, watch TV, listen to the radio, or read. These activities distract your senses from the food you are eating and from observing and responding to the promptings of your body.
- Stop eating when your body is satiated.

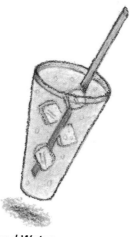

Iced Water
Iced water inhibits digestion, which leads to the production of ama and disturbances of the doshas. As Dr. Vasant Lad says "Ice is not nice".

THE CONSUMER

The individual factors to consider in order to assess the right diet for you are:
- *Your constitution (see pp. 38-41)*
- *Any current doshic imbalances (see pp. 62-3)*
- *Age (see p. 10)*
- *The strength of your digestion (see pp. 49-50)*
- *Your lifestyle*

CONSIDERING CHANGES TO YOUR DIET

Deciding on a diet that is right for you is often the hardest part about using Ayurvedic principles. There is no easy answer, but it is important not to make quick or dramatic changes. This gives you time to learn about the doshic classification of foods (see pp. 133-43) and to become more aware of the effects your current diet may have. Then, if you make one small change at a time, you will experience for yourself how foods affect your wellbeing.

The changes may involve eating different foods, different combinations of foods, or preparing foods by different methods. If you propose using different food items then you need to consider ways that these can be incorporated into your diet. Generally, it is not easy to give up foods you eat habitually, and you will find it hard initially to think of suitable alternatives. Your digestive system will have adapted to the foods you eat, and sudden or big changes will act as a shock to the system and may lead to digestive or other problems. Make gradual changes over weeks and months.

Pacifying the Doshas
The lists below summarize the main rules for each dosha-pacifying diet. In addition, you should choose foods from the YES column of the food charts to pacify that dosha (see pp. 133-43) and avoid those in the NO column. Occasional lapses will not hurt, it is what you do habitually that matters.

PACIFYING PITTA	
YES	NO
Eat salads	Avoid sour, salty, spicy foods
Use only cooling herbs and spices	Avoid alcohol
	Avoid meat
	Avoid fried foods

PACIFYING VATA	
YES	NO
Use spices	Avoid raw foods
Eat heavy, warm, oily, moist foods	Avoid dry foods
Have regular meal times	Avoid leafy vegetables
	Avoid cold foods
	Avoid frozen foods

PACIFYING KAPHA	
YES	NO
Eat plenty of vegetables	Avoid sweet and salty foods
Eat salads	Avoid dairy products
Eat dry, light foods	Avoid fried foods
Use spices	Avoid frozen foods

WHICH PACIFYING DIET?

Once you know your constitution (see pp. 38-41), then you can select foods that tend to pacify your predominant dosha, since this is the dosha that tends to increase most easily. Pacifying your predominant dosha allows you to gain increased vitality by producing a better balance of doshic energy than exists in your constitutional balance. Before you follow a pacifying diet for your predominant dosha, check your other doshas are in balance (see p. 63).

If you have a duo-type constitution, you need a diet that does not increase either of your predominant doshas. For example, if you have a pitta–kapha constitution you should select foods that will not excessively increase pitta or kapha. In addition, you will have to make seasonal adjustments, so that a pitta-pacifying diet will be appropriate in the pitta season (summer) and a kapha-pacifying diet in winter.

Selection of Diet
Look at the lists below to identify your doshic state and then follow the appropriate diet indicated at the top of the column. For instance, if you have a vata constitution with increased pitta, follow a pitta-pacifying diet. To discover which foods suit which diets, see the food charts on pages 133-43.

Vata-pacifying Diet for:
- *Vata constitution with no increased dosha*
- *Vata constitution with increased vata*
- *Pitta constitution with increased vata (but do not increase pitta)*
- *Kapha constitution with increased vata (but do not increase kapha)*

Kapha-pacifying Diet for:
- *Kapha constitution with no increased dosha*
- *Kapha constitution with increased kapha*
- *Vata constitution with increased kapha (but do not increase vata)*
- *Pitta constitution with increased kapha (but do not increase pitta)*

Pitta-pacifying Diet for:
- *Pitta constitution with no increased dosha*
- *Pitta constitution with increased pitta*
- *Vata constitution with increased pitta (but do not increase vata)*
- *Kapha constitution with increased pitta (but do not increase kapha)*

However, if one of your non-predominant doshas is excessive (see p. 63), then follow a diet that pacifies the excessive dosha until that dosha has returned to your constitutional norm. At the same time, try to avoid increasing your predominant dosha. Follow the advice given for people with duo-type constitutions above. For example, if you have a pitta constitution but your vata is excessive, follow a vata-pacifying diet, but avoid eating too many foods that increase pitta. Monitor the signs of excess doshas in your mind and body (see p. 63) and when the excess vata has been eliminated, follow a pitta-pacifying diet.

Preparing Food for a Family

If everyone in your household follows the same dosha-pacifying diet then whoever organizes the meals can plan menus around the appropriate ingredients and principles. But if you all have differing doshic requirements, planning an appropriate menu can be complicated. Do not try to change the meals until you feel familiar with the general principles – providing a diet suitable for everyone will seem impossible to start with unless you cook separate meals!

Before you make any changes, classify the foods you buy into vata, pitta, and kapha. If you intend to pacify two doshas, look for items in the food charts (see pp. 133-43) that apply to both, and substitute these where possible. There is no easy solution, but moderation and individual use of condiments and garnishes will help. The selection of suitable side dishes in Indian cooking is a very useful way to make a tri-doshically balanced meal. Another way is to use one-pot cooking as often as possible (see p. 146).

As your understanding of Ayurveda grows, so too will your confidence in preparing balanced meals. Remember, food is to be enjoyed so do not let anxieties about getting it right spoil your meals. Strong digestion, clear perceptions, good company, and fresh food cooked with love allow you to experience the natural deliciousness of food and satisfaction in body and mind.

Garnishes
You can add garnishes individually according to dosha: for example, pittas can add cilantro or coriander leaves, mint, raita (yogurt-based condiment), or shredded coconut; vatas and kaphas can add fresh ground pepper or ginger pickle.

FOOD PROFILES

Vicky's Diet (p. 112)

Vicky is a vegetarian with a vata constitution and a vata imbalance. She also has toxins due to her incapacity to digest fully improper food combinations. She should eat regularly and simply, and in particular avoid raw and dry foods. She should select foods from the vata-pacifying (YES) column of the food charts (see pp. 133-43).

Giles' Diet (p. 81)

Giles has a kapha constitution and his favourite foods tend to increase kapha. He should avoid fried, dairy, and sugary foods, and select foods from the kapha-pacifying (YES) column of the food charts (see pp. 133-43).

Martin's Diet (pp. 105, 182-3)

Martin has a pitta constitution and excess pitta. His current pitta-increasing diet should be altered to reduce pitta. He should avoid fried foods, alcohol, and coffee, and cut down on meat, especially red meat. He should select foods from the pitta-pacifying (YES) column of the food charts (see pp. 133-43).

VICKY'S DIET

Meal	Summary of Diet from Weekly Diet Record	Suggestions to Adjust Diet to Help Pacify Vata
Breakfast	Oat-based muesli with dried fruit, cold milk, and yogurt. Boiled egg with toast. Coffee.	Cooked oats. Eat fruits separately, and soak dried fruits. Do not mix milk and yogurt. Scrambled eggs.
Lunch	Salads of lettuce, tomatoes, and cucumber, with quiche or cheese and baked potato.	Vegetables sautéed or steamed. Replace hard cheese with cottage cheese. Use freshly ground black pepper. Eat sweet potato or cook white potato with oil and spices. Whole wheat macaroni and sauce. Lassi.
Evening meal	Lentil, bean, or nut dishes with salad or vegetables. Rice pudding. Yogurt, cheesecake, or fruit.	Limit use of legumes to mung beans, some soya products, and red lentils. Use cumin, coriander, and fennel in bean dishes to help reduce gases and their tendency to cause constipation. Try kitcheri with bread or chapattis and pickle. Have lassi in place of yogurt. Eat fruit as snacks on its own.
Snacks	Rice cakes, chocolate. Occasional alcoholic drink, apple juice, carbonated water.	Sweet fruits. Wholewheat or oatmeal cookies with spices, e.g. cinnamon and ginger. Ginger tea, hot spiced milk. Small amount of alcohol to stimulate the appetite.

GILES' DIET

Meal	Summary of Diet from Weekly Diet Record	Suggestions to Adjust Diet to Help Pacify Kapha
Breakfast	Sugar-coated cereals with cold milk. Toast with butter and jam. Coffee. At weekends, a cooked breakfast with fried bacon, eggs, tomatoes, and bread.	A light breakfast before 7.30 am of muesli (without wheat) and drink juice, such as apple, instead of cold milk.
Lunch	Cheese sandwiches or pizza or scampi and chips. Danish pastry or other dessert. Beer.	Soups or salads, but with very little oil-based dressing. Lassi.
Evening meal	Pies, e.g. steak and kidney, or roast beef or chicken, with boiled or roasted vegetables. Likes dessert most days, sometimes with cream.	Freshwater fish or chicken, steamed vegetables. Dishes with basmati rice or millet. Baked apples with clove and cinnamon.
Snacks	Chocolate biscuits, tea, squashes, and fizzy drinks.	Fruit. Apple juice, grape juice, herb teas.

MARTIN'S DIET

Meal	Summary of Diet from Weekly Diet Record	Suggestions to Adjust Diet to Help Pacify Pitta
Breakfast	If away from home, fried breakfast. Coffee. At home, coffee and skips breakfast. More coffee and whatever is to hand on arrival at office.	Have breakfast. Oatmeal, shredded wheat, toast, or pancakes.
Lunch	Sandwich unless having business lunch often at Italian or Mexican restaurants. Wine.	Stick to the salad bars. Do not have alcohol.
Evening meal	A large variety of different foods, often steaks. Likes tasty sauces, especially those with tomatoes, garlic, onions, or chilli. Wine and liqueurs.	Rice dishes and pasta. Have herb sauces in place of spicy ones. Reduce the amount of alcohol.
Snacks	Salty snacks. Coffee. Spirits.	Sweet fruits. Cold drinks, dilute sweet fruit juices, mint tea.

SPICES AND HERBS

In Western cookery, spices and herbs are used in small amounts, mainly for flavoring. Ayurveda has a wider approach. In addition to adding deliciousness to food, spices and herbs stimulate the appetite and aid digestion, by increasing secretion of digestive juices, by increasing absorption in the intestines, by reducing gases, and by influencing the doshas. There are some spices that should be in every home. If you have not tried cooking with spices before, the ten that follow will give you a good foundation.

The energetics (see pp. 52-3) of each herb and spice is shown – either heating or cooling. The spices also affect the doshas, either by increasing (I) or pacifying (P); the effect is given in the order on V, P, and then K.

Black Pepper
Heating   P* I P
Increases appetite and agni. Aids the digestion of dairy products. Too much will cause irritation and dryness. Use freshly ground.

Coriander
Cooling   P P P
Helps counteract the effects of pungent foods. Eases gases and generally tones the digestive system. Use whole seed or powdered. Use leaves as a garnish.

Turmeric
Heating   P* P* P
Strengthens digestion and generally improves metabolism. Aids the digestion of protein. The root is used ground. Widely used in Indian cooking, giving dishes a yellow color. It can stain clothes, work surfaces, and china.

Cardamom
Heating   P P* P
Kindles agni without increasing pitta, unless used in excess. Reduces the mucus-forming effects of dairy products. Use in coffee to counter some effects of caffeine. Use powdered or whole seeds.

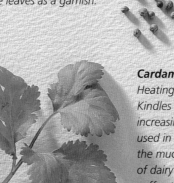

P = pacifies I = increases * = Pacifies unless used in excess

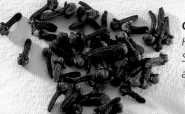

Cinnamon

Heating P P* P
Stimulates agni. Is less like-
ly than ginger to affect
pitta. Use powdered,
sticks, or pieces.

Clove

Heating P I P
Stimulates agni and helps with
absorption. Use whole or ground.

Cumin

Slightly heating P P* P
Pacifies vata and kapha with-
out increasing pitta unless used
in excess. Helps reduce ama
and gases and tones the diges-
tive system. Use the seeds
whole or powdered.

Ginger

Heating P I P
Highly regarded in Ayurveda. Works on all tis-
sues, especially digestive and respiratory.
Stimulates agni, helps relieve gases and consti-
pation, and vata or kapha indigestion. Do not
use if there is high pitta, temperature, bleeding
conditions, or ulcers. Use root, either fresh or
dried. Fresh is best for vata and dried for kapha.

Fennel

Cooling P P P
Increases agni without increasing
pitta. Helps prevent gases. Either
chew the seeds after a meal or
add to vegetables that tend to
produce gas when cooking. Use
seeds, whole or powdered.

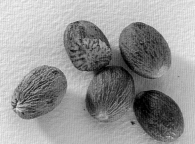

Nutmeg

Heating P I P
Helps with absorption. Is calm-
ing. Use ground and sparingly.

Drinks from Herbs and Spices

Be flexible in your use of herbs and spices; select them according to your needs and to the seasons. If you have a lot of heat in your body (for example, those with a pitta constitution or excess pitta), then hot, pungent spices will not be good for you. However, you can use black pepper, cardamom, cinnamon, and turmeric in moderation (see pp. 158-9). Coriander and fennel are cooling and therefore beneficial for you. People with a naturally cold make-up (those with vata or kapha constitutions) can use all spices. The heating ones, such as ginger, black pepper, and clove are especially useful in the winter months. Whatever your constitution, make sure your kitchen contains a selection of spices.

A good way for you to become familiar with the taste and effects of spices and herbs is to make drinks from them. Enjoy making your own teas according to your specific requirements, and drink them as alternatives to the usual tea or coffee. Here are some recipes for various drinks which you can try. The amounts given are a guide; adjust them to your own preferences.

Ginger Tea
This very warming drink can be made with fresh or dried ginger. For one mug, use EITHER about a teaspoon of grated or finely chopped fresh ginger OR a flat quarter tea-spoon of dried ginger. Then add boiling water. Let it steep for five minutes. Strain before drinking. Add honey or brown sugar if desired.

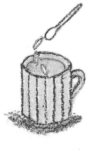

Heating Drink
A mixture of five ground spices, this is easiest to prepare in small batches and then store in a jar. The proportions are one part black pepper and four parts each of cardamom, cinnamon, clove, and ginger. Experiment to see if these are your favoured proportions, but beware of overdoing the black pepper or it will dominate. Mix these together until they are well blended. You can make a simple tea using a flat quarter teaspoon of the mixture per mug and then

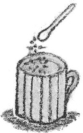

adding hot water; let it brew for a few minutes. Add honey or brown sugar if desired when the drink has brewed. You could also add a couple of pinches of this mixture to a cup of ordinary tea – just for a change.

Cooling Drink

This tea is cooling in its energetic properties rather than its temperature and is good for all constitutional types. It is made with equal proportions of the seeds of cumin, coriander, and fennel. Allow one teaspoon of seeds per mug. Add hot water and allow to brew before straining and drinking. An easy way to make this tea is to mix a batch of the seeds, store them in a jar, and use a mesh tea ball for the seeds when you need a drink.

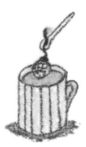

Spiced Milk

To a small mug, add generous pinches (such as a quarter teaspoon) of ground ginger, cardamom, and cinnamon, and a small pinch of nutmeg. Fill with hot milk. When it has cooled slightly, add honey to taste if desired. Stir well. This makes a good bedtime drink, soothing vata and encouraging sleep. You can try different proportions or spices, such as clove in place of the cinnamon.

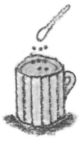

Lassi

This drink changes the natural properties of yogurt and is recommended at the end of a meal to help digestion. Adjust the spices according to your constitution. Vata and kapha types could have cumin, ginger, cardamom, and/or black pepper. The black pepper will give it a kick, so use with care. Pitta types should choose coriander or fennel. Blend equal parts of yogurt and water and add, in total, a half to one teaspoon of your chosen spices. Mix in a small amount of sweetener, such as honey or maple syrup, if you so desire.

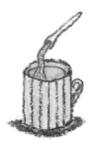

KITCHERI

Kitcheri is a one-pot dish made with rice, beans, spices, and often with vegetables. You can adapt the spices and vegetables to your tastes and doshic needs. Nutritious and very easy to digest, kitcheri is recommended for irregular digestion (see pp. 76-7). If you use rice in the proportion of two to one with beans, the amount of protein available to the body will be more than if the rice and beans are eaten separately. If you have low digestive strength, kitcheri should be cooked to the consistency of mashed potatoes.

Ingredients:
Oil	Spices
Basmati rice	Split yellow mung beans
Water	Vegetables

You can vary your choice of spices and also the amounts you use. Initially, try half a teaspoon per person of cumin, coriander, and fennel seeds and half a teaspoon of turmeric powder. This will make a dish suitable for all constitutional types. For a warmer kitcheri, add ginger.

For each person, allow a handful of Basmati rice (about 1oz or 30g) and half as much split yellow mung beans. Mix rice and beans together and wash in cold water.

In a pan, melt one tablespoon of ghee or oil and add the seeds. Cook for a minute. Then add the ground spices and washed grains and beans, stirring them to coat with the oil. Add sufficient hot water to cover the grains and beans by about 2in (5cm), bring to the boil and simmer gently, stirring occasionally. Make sure the pan does not become dry and add more water as required.

Add diced vegetables if you like – root ones with the rice, and leafy or softer ones nearer the end of the cooking time. Select vegetables that are appropriate for your doshas (see food charts on pp. 133-43). The dish is cooked when the rice is soft and a grain easily squashes between thumb and forefinger. Most of the liquid should have been absorbed or evaporated. Kitcheri can be served with chapattis. Pitta types could use coriander leaves as a garnish. Vata and kapha types can have some pickle.

A One-pot Dish
Kitcheri, a rice and bean dish, is nutritious and easy both to prepare and to digest. As a note of caution, kitcheri may cause constipation if eaten regularly. Adding diced vegetables will prevent this (see main text).

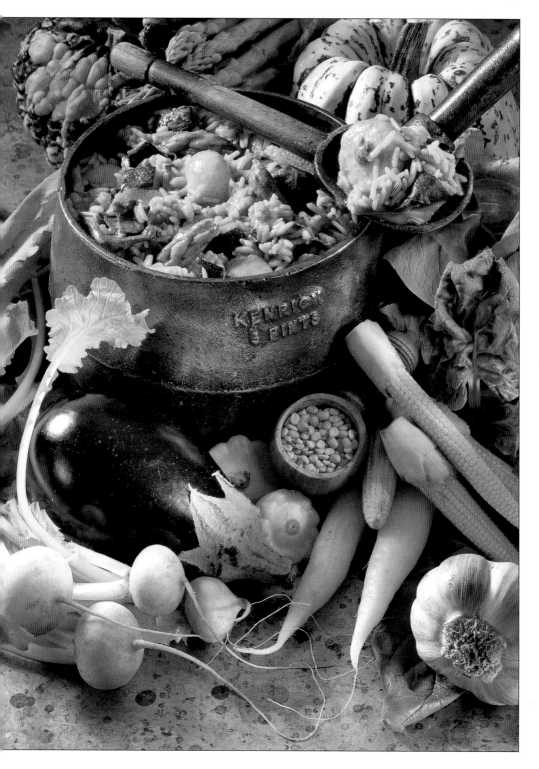

EATING VEGETABLES

Vegetables should form 20% to 40% of your diet. If you have a kapha constitution eat plenty of vegetables because generally they are light.

Ayurveda does not recommend eating raw vegetables because they are rough and hard to digest. However, they are fine on occasions if your digestion is good. Salads are better in summer than winter as they pacify pitta but increase vata. If you are in the vata age (over 55) eat salads only occasionally, and with an oil dressing. Raw tomatoes disturb all the doshas, so avoid eating them regularly. Raw vegetables take longer to digest than cooked ones so try not to mix them in the same meal.

When deciding how to cook your vegetables, think of the qualities the cooking will add. If you stir fry or sauté vegetables, the oil will increase kapha and pitta but not vata. If the vegetables are only lightly cooked and are still crunchy, they will still tend to increase vata and be harder to digest.

Potatoes are vata-genic and baking dries them further. The "jacket" adds another vata quality – roughness – and is hard to digest. So enjoy baked potatoes when your vata is not aggravated. You can reduce the vata-genic qualities of potatoes by cooking them in the way suggested on page 165. Steaming vegetables preserves their flavour as well as making them easier to digest.

As far as possible, buy organic vegetables that are in season and locally grown or, even better, eat ones you or your friends have grown with love.

Fresh Vegetables
Enjoy the flavours and freshness of recently picked, locally grown vegetables. Select ones that are suitable for your doshas.

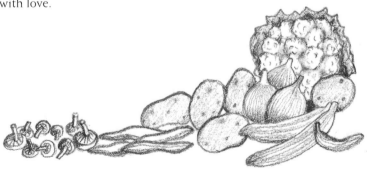

Cooking diced vegetables with spices in a small amount of water is suitable for all doshic types. You can experiment with different combinations of spices and vegetables. Select one or more vegetables that are suitable for your doshic requirements (see food charts pp. 133-43). Wash them and cut them into bite-size pieces. A little creative chopping adds to the visual appearance of the dish.

Use a large, heavy-bottomed, preferably stainless steel, shallow pan with a lid. Over a moderate heat, add 2–3 tablespoons of oil – do not overdo the oil if you have a kapha constitution. Then add your chosen spices. Select them to benefit your agni and doshas (see pp. 158-9) but also for their aromas and flavours. If spices are new to you, start with half a teaspoon each of cumin seeds and mustard seeds – black mustard seeds are stronger than yellow ones.

If you use whole seeds, put them in the oil and cook them until they begin to pop. Then add your selection of ground spices (e.g. turmeric or fennel), and cook for a moment before adding the chopped vegetables. Stir the vegetables for a minute to coat them in the spices and oil, and then add a small amount of water.

Bring to the boil, put the lid on, and turn down to a low to moderate heat until the vegetables are cooked. The amount of water needed depends on the type of vegetables you are cooking – root vegetables need more than softer vegetables, such as courgettes – and the size you have cut them. Essentially, the aim is to leave no excess water when the vegetables are ready to eat (you can add more water if necessary during the cooking).

Kitcheri and vegetables cooked in this way, with garnishes suitable for your doshas (see p. 155) and chapattis or other flat bread followed by a glass of lassi (see p. 161) makes an easily digestible, nutritious, tasty, and inexpensive meal that is balanced for all doshas.

Mind and Emotions

यद्गुणं चाभीक्षणं पुरुषमनुवर्तते सत्त्वं
तत्सत्त्वमेवोपदिशन्ति मुनयो बाहुल्यानुशयात् ॥

According to the Acharyas the mind of a person is qualified on the basis of the type of
his repeated action; it is so because that quality must be predominating in him.
(Charaka Samhita *Chapter 8: 6)*

The perfect human being experiences no disturbances in
energy flow, since all levels function in harmony. Body,
senses, mind, consciousness, and those parts of us that are
beyond description, together express the wonder and
beauty of life. Disturbances at any level can affect health.

Your body, the most accessible part of your being, is a
reflection of the less tangible parts of you; an expression of
all your experiences and how you have assimilated them.
Your body requires proper care, which may be lacking as
the everyday mind continuously seeks fresh experiences.

Ayurveda teaches that the everyday mind has qualities,
and therefore must be physical, though more subtle than
the body. Like the body, it has to be balanced to function
properly. The mind is faster and more demanding than the
body, and thus harder to bring under proper control.
Ahamkara (see pp. 18-21) may identify with itself so
strongly that the link with your inner wisdom appears lost,
along with the unity of being part, with all others, of cosmic consciousness.

According to Ayurveda, all illnesses are psychosomatic. Both mind and body are involved and should be considered in restoring health and maintaining wellness, as benefits at one level of being will be reflected at other levels.

The Everyday Mind

Your everyday mind and ordinary intellect link your senses and actions. They regulate the interfaces between your external and internal environments, and the changes that happen internally. Your mind pervades your whole body.

Everything we experience on the physical level comes via one or more of our senses. All our perceptions have qualities related to VPK. This is most easily demonstrated with taste (see pp. 54-5), but it applies to other senses as well. A violent film, for example, has pitta-aggravating qualities. Tickling enhances vata.

You cannot be conscious of every sensation you receive, but remember that the qualities of sensations may increase your doshas according to the principle of "like increases like". So limit your exposure to those qualities you do not want, but enjoy those that will add to your wellbeing.

The clarity of your mind is affected by how you use it. Like a muscle, it needs the right kind of use and neither too little nor too much. Pitta types tend to have sharp, quick minds – they love reading and doing mental puzzles – which they easily overuse. Kaphas are slower thinkers who generally would benefit from more mental stimulation than they are used to. Vatas dream up projects, and have new schemes every time you meet them. They need to concentrate on one or two of their sound ideas, in order to move forward into the planning and execution stages.

Whatever your constitution, too much intellectual work aggravates pitta. Too much sensory stimulation, such as watching TV and VDUs, disturbs vata. Boring, repetitive tasks dull the mind and increase kapha. What is "too much" depends on the individual and their current circumstances.

Emotional Eating

We usually eat sweet foods when we crave comfort. Comfort foods often have kapha qualities in both their taste and texture. As you heal your emotional hurts, use senses other than taste to give yourself comfort and nurturing, such as the company of friends, an aromatherapy massage, or relaxing music.

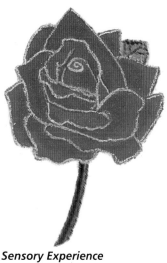

Sensory Experience

The smell of a rose is sweet, a quality associated with kapha.

UNDERSTANDING EMOTIONS

Those who express their emotions often feel that this is better than suppressing them. Ayurveda says it is better to understand emotions rather than suppressing or expressing them. In understanding them, they are transformed and released. If you are angry, look behind the events that triggered your anger. Then look behind the anger. Behind anger, or fear, and other negative emotions there is usually a hurt. A deep, deep hurt that you have tried to silence.

Deep unresolved emotions can disturb the mind. They suck your energy to parts seemingly beyond your control or manifest themselves as illness in the body. You may not be able to resolve all emotional pains as they occur, particularly if an event overwhelms you or if emotional traumas happen before you have the maturity to digest and assimilate them.

The body and mind have powerful survival instincts which can override conscious processes. Phobias, or less clearly labelled but equally inappropriate and habitual actions, may be behaviours set up as defence or denial mechanisms. The problem of the phobia diverts attention from the unresolved hurt. Energy is used to maintain the denial or avoidance rather than for creating wellness.

The resolution of pain releases the energy used in denial or avoidance, or that manifests as physical symptoms. Take time to resolve your emotional pains. It is a process of small steps forward, and some seemingly backward until at the right time you experience the change inside. The change comes through understanding, acceptance, and letting go.

Contacting your inner wisdom (see p. 174) helps when you are trying to resolve your deep emotional hurts. Observe your body and mind as you enquire about what you are experiencing. Ask yourself why you are experiencing this. Let your connection with your inner wisdom grow, and let it show you your unique way to understanding. Open yourself to the inner guidance that is always ready to reveal the opportunities you truly need. You have to have awareness to see them. Then it is vital to act upon them.

Coming through Pain
Emotional hurts can be very painful and you may feel unwilling to face that pain. Coming through emotional pain is one way to release it. It is generally acknowledged, for example, that the only way to resolve the pain of bereavement is to come through it. If the grieving process stops before the pain is resolved then different psychological and physical problems arise, which may not be seen as connected to the bereavement. Apply this principle of "coming through pain" to all types of pain you experience.

Start by seeing coincidences or synchronistic events in your life. Ask yourself simple questions as if a wise person were listening to you. Immediate or direct answers are not necessarily given. As you go about your daily life something may happen that seems coincidental. Someone may say something or give you a book that has something that strikes a chord in you, or you meet someone who opens new ideas about your internal questions. The circumstances of these coincidences are unique to each individual, and easily dismissed by the logical mind. However, use common sense and discrimination, but do not miss the quiet way in which the guidance comes. This gets easier with practice, and in time you will find yourself becoming more and more in flow with your life.

You may be guided to seek support from someone as you come to understand and acknowledge all you experienced, how you reacted at the time, and how you have been affected. When this inner acknowledgment comes, you will feel the force that held the pain dissolving. You are ready to assimilate the good squeezed from the pain.

Love Yourself

The release is a process, a means by which we grow. Take it in small sips. Remember to love yourself through all this. Your mind and body always strive toward health, but their starting point is how they are now. They need time, nurturing, routine, and gentle discipline.

EXPLORING YOUR PAIN

When you experience pain, either emotional or physical, or you have an emotional problem, take time to stop and see how you think about the pain or problem as well as taking practical steps to alleviate it.

Watch and experience the pain dispassionately with an enquiring mind. Relate the qualities of your experiences to the doshas (see pp. 30-1, 75, 78). Ask yourself questions about what you are experiencing. Be patient; it usually requires practice to obtain the insights. Learn to recognize your way of knowing that you have received a meaningful insight. Trust yourself to receive the counsel of your inner wisdom, which may be hidden by the chatter of the everyday mind.

You can do this enquiring, observation exercise with any problems in your life. Be with the problem and explore all its facets. Remember, you are the observer. Lovingly, patiently, diligently search for the keys to understanding and resolution.

LIFE EVENTS AND CHANGE

Traumas and life events, even good ones, affect our health because change aggravates vata. Vata is the most volatile of the doshas; according to ancient texts, over 50% of illness is due to vata disturbances. Many symptoms of stress in modern life are due to excess vata. Take extra care of yourself at times of change, to prevent vata imbalance. Try to understand how your doshas are affected by change and life's events, and how they affect your reactions to them. And try to see times of ill health or stress as indicators of the adjustments required in your lifestyle.

Major life events include changes in both family circumstances (e.g. divorce, marriage, pregnancy, childbirth, children leaving home) and working life (a new job/ boss, redundancy, retirement, moving to a new location). The death of someone we love leaves us empty (vata), but other emotions may be bound up in the pain: for example, anger (pitta) at the circumstances of the death, or difficulty in letting go (kapha).

Assessing Life Events

Use these headings to assess the major events in your life:
• Description of the event
• Duration of the event
• Season when the event took place
• Effects of the event on your body
• Thoughts and emotions experienced

Think about the qualitative effects on your mind and body. Relate these to the qualities of VPK (see pp. 28-31, 37) and to emotions (see p. 36, 78, 168-9) in order to assess the doshic effects of your experiences.

Compare the chronological order of your life events with previous ailments or illnesses, and use the ailment assessment (see p. 80) to understand which excess dosha manifested the symptoms. This helps build the picture of the doshic patterns in your life and to show tendencies in the way you react. Ask an empathetic friend to help you.

A Newborn Baby

The arrival of a new human being signals many changes in a family. All doshas can be affected by the physical and emotional experiences. Vata, in particular, will be increased by the birth process itself, by the change in routine, and by the interruption to, and loss of, sleep.

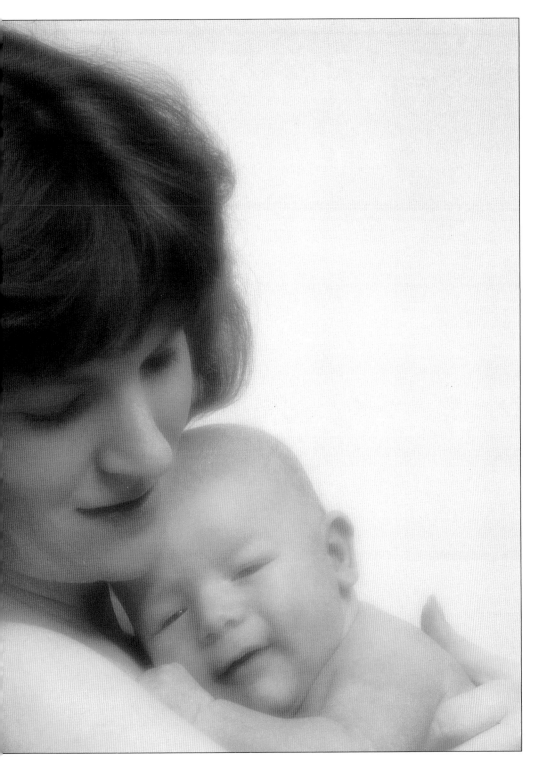

REPRESSED EMOTIONS AND THE BODY

We have seen that negative emotions and repressing emotions aggravate the doshas (see pp. 78, 168-9). Unresolved emotions can also cause weak spots (see p. 70), which show no symptoms unless the doshas are aggravated and spread into the tissue types. Massage can reach the seven tissue types, which according to Ayurveda are connected to the layers of the skin.

Massage is known to improve metabolism and to have other physiological effects; and, in the right conditions, massage can help release repressed emotions. This takes time, and the environment must be safe, physically and emotionally. Also, the masseur's touch and manner must be caring and sensitive. In these conditions you have the opportunity to be with and let go of repressed emotions, but only when you are ready to release them. Tears are a sign that the body is cleansing emotions. Always be gentle and loving toward yourself. Trust what you are experiencing. Never force anything. It has taken time to become as you are and time will be needed to change.

Negative Emotions

Dr. Vasant Lad teaches that certain negative emotions have an affinity with some organs (see table below). All experiences are impressed on the memory of muscle tissues. Within Ayurveda's understanding of the body there are specific connections between certain emotions and muscles, and between those muscles and certain organs. The layers of skin are related to the seven levels of tissue; thus all the tissues can be affected by massage.

ORGANS AND NEGATIVE EMOTIONS

ORGAN	EMOTION
Adrenals	Anxiety, sense of lack of support
Bladder	Insecurity
Colon	Nervousness
Heart	Sense of lack of love, feelings of deep hurt
Lungs	Sadness and grief
Kidney	Fear
Gallbladder	Hate
Liver	Anger
Small intestine	Sense of failure
Spleen	Greed, attachment, possessiveness
Stomach	Lack of fulfilment, lack of contentment

RELATIONSHIPS

Life is relationships. Your wellbeing affects and is affected by your relationships with yourself, your body, your pains, your thoughts, your emotions, your partner, your family, your friends, your colleagues, your work, your leisure activities, and your environment.

When your relationship with yourself is right the rest will move into balance. The key is to love yourself, which means accepting yourself just as you are. In loving yourself you are able to love the rest of creation. You reflect what you are. Awareness of who you really are and understanding of your uniqueness will allow you to love yourself. By loving yourself, you will give yourself the time needed for the welfare of your body and mind and spirit.

Through learning to love yourself, you will also come to respect yourself. You will also find the resources within that allow you to make adjustments to your attitudes and your life, which will help to bring your other relationships into balance. If you find your place in the dance of creation, it helps those around you find their places, too.

Some situations in life do not seem to find proper resolution, and you may have to face hard decisions and painful acceptance. Not accepting a situation, having regrets over your actions, or not feeling able to act, all take energy and can affect your physical health.

The qualities of the emotions in your relationships affect your doshas. If there is much anger, pitta increases. Fear deranges vata. Possessiveness affects kapha. As you deal with difficult times, look after your physical health by taking practical steps through your diet and lifestyle to keep your doshas balanced.

Meditation and awareness (see pp. 176-7) will help you understand your relationships. Learn to be the observer. See what is happening, but do not judge. Many human communications are clouded by the filters of past hurts and judgmental attitudes.

SPACE TO GROW

When your doshas are balanced, positive aspects are naturally expressed in all your relationships. For example, communication (vata), attention (pitta), and support and compassion (kapha). This brings space, allowing all your relationships to grow and develop. The space gives room for unconditional love, the energy of the universe, and the source of healing.

INDIVIDUAL IDENTITY

Inappropriate opinions and judgments, or the harbouring of deep hurts, can bring a sense of isolation, separation, or division. We lose the awareness that we are a part of universal creation and cannot be separate from it. We take our hurts and pains personally, when we forget that we share in the pain, and also the joys, of humanity.

Modern pressures make it hard to remain connected with "who we really are", especially if we identify ourselves as only our emotions, thoughts, everyday mind, and physical body. When we acknowledge hidden levels of our being we touch our inner wisdom and come to know "who we really are" – the experiencer experiencing existence.

It is important to have a strong individual identity, or ahamkara (see pp. 18-21), so we are not open to unwelcome influences. In building our identity, the mind may want to gain power and perpetuate itself, rather than be a servant of "who we really are". This is subtle, but we can end up defining ourselves as our own strong attitudes and opinions. If this happens we forget "who we really are" and lose the awareness of how and why the attitudes were formed, and whether they are still relevant for our wellbeing.

This is a very difficult and often painful part of ourselves to look at. For most of us it strikes at what we regard as the core of our being. Courage is needed to examine and, perhaps, change these structures of our minds. Often, they are self-made filters that colour and weaken our connection with "who we really are" and cause us to act in ways that prevent us realizing our full potential.

Identity with deep attitudes does not change easily. Ask yourself why you think as you do about issues affecting your wellbeing. Do your opinions help you obtain the best outcome, or would a change in your approach open up greater possibilities? If you find yourself resisting change, ask yourself why, but without being critical. Change should only happen at the appropriate time. Gradual change is preferable and less distressing than sudden change.

Integration
Regular meditation, or stilling the mind, allows the gradual integration of all aspects of your being.

WHO AM I?

This is a question that has no answer. But if asked in stillness or meditation it brings growing awareness of parts of your being that are beyond words – insights of "who you really are". It heals internal wounds and brings integration. Everyone experiences this in different ways. As you continue to ask "Who am I?" your inner wisdom will grow whatever your outer circumstances, and a light will shine through any pains you still have to bear.

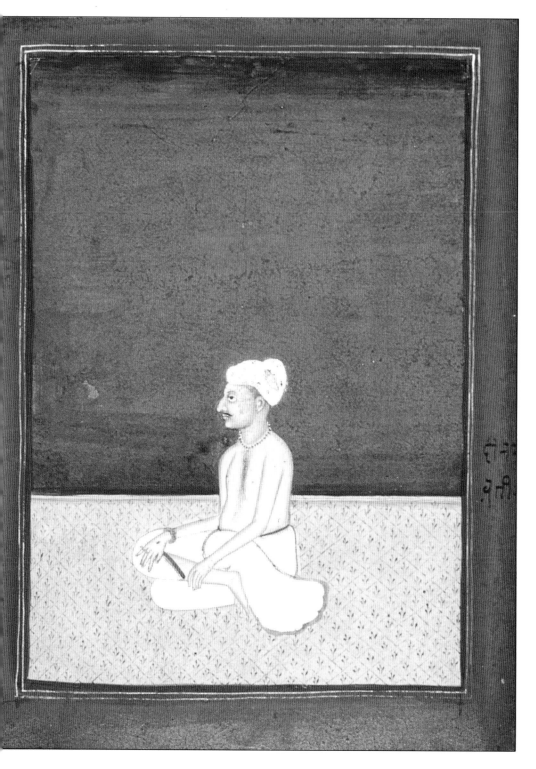

AWARENESS AND MEDITATION

Meditation maintains mental and emotional health by allowing you to be aware of "who you really are". If you already meditate then continue as usual, otherwise the first step is to practise stilling the everyday mind (see below). When you first start, many questions arise: how should you meditate correctly, what are you trying to achieve, or how can you understand what you experience? Let the questions pass, without worrying or trying to answer them. Give yourself a regular quiet time when you can become aware of your inner wisdom, which can guide all aspects of your life.

Life is Meditation

Meditation can be more than spending 10 minutes every morning and evening letting your mind be still, although this in itself is important. You can live your whole life as a meditation, as the observer witnessing your life. You are vital, aware of how your thoughts and actions affect your wellbeing and the wellbeing of those around you.

Living life in this state of awareness is a skill that needs practice until it becomes part of you. Start by taking a few moments (at different times during the day) consciously to observe how your body is feeling. Do this at any time – at the bus stop, at your desk, while driving, or preparing a meal. Are both sides of your body balanced or are you putting more weight on one side? Adjust your posture if

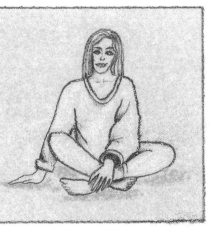

....STILLING THE EVERYDAY MIND....

If meditation is new to you, here is a simple way to learn to still the mind. Make yourself comfortable, preferably sitting on the floor or a chair. Sit with your spine upright but relaxed. Focus your attention on your breath. Observe it going in and coming out. Do not change how you are breathing, just watch. On the inhalation silently say "SO", and on the exhalation "HUM". When you notice that the mind has wandered away from the breath, gently bring it back and continue with "SO-HUM".

necessary, but do not worry if a few moments later you are back in your habitual position. Do you have tension or aches in any part of your body – for example, in your shoulders or legs? If you do, do not make a judgment about that or yourself; just gently move the tense muscles or rub the aches, and carry on with what you are doing.

Consciously note the state of your everyday mind. Is that little voice chattering away in your head, repeating judgments from the past and worries about the future? Is the chattering interfering with your mind's clarity, clouding your perceptions and actions now? That little voice is one of the hardest things to control. Become aware of the tone of its chatter. It can act like brainwashing. Often, these repetitive thoughts are unloving and critical of yourself. Even if you cannot turn it off you can change the record so that it has positive and loving messages. Every time you catch yourself thinking negative thoughts, cancel them mentally and create a positive thought. A regular 10 minutes' quiet time really helps quieten the mind.

As you learn more about Ayurveda and the doshas, you will find you put your awareness increasingly into your daily activities. You use the qualitative way of thinking to see what is happening around and within you, and then make conscious instead of habitual choices.

> ❝ *Meditation is one of the most serious things. You can do it all day, in the office, with the family, when you say to someone, "I love you", when you are considering your children.... And when you so meditate you will find in it an extraordinary beauty; you will act rightly at every moment; and if you do not act rightly at a given moment it does not matter, you will pick it up again – you will not waste time in regret. Meditation is part of life not something different from life.*
>
> *Krishnamurti,* Meditation

Making Changes

क्रमेणापचिता दोषाः क्रमेणोपचिता गुणाः ।
सन्तो यान्त्यपुनर्भावमप्रकम्प्या भवन्ति च ॥

*The bad effects diminished gradually and the good effects increased gradually,
attain (the state of) non-recurrence and become stable.*
(Astanga Hrdayam *Chapter 7: 50)*

You need to apply Ayurveda in your life to experience its
benefits. Before this can happen, you need to take many
factors into account. And as you examine the qualities in
your life more closely, you find that the doshic influences
are not always clear cut, making it confusing which dosha
you need to pacify. You end up thinking you need to pacify
them all! So where do you begin?

First have confidence and trust yourself. You already feel
and think in qualities; now you can begin to use qualitative
information in logical and intuitive ways. You know your
mind and body very well, though often your inner wisdom
may seem obscured by habits detrimental to your health.

The very first step to maintaining good health is to
make sure you have good digestion (see p. 179). This prevents ama (see p. 77) and builds healthy tissues, which
results in sufficient ojas (see p. 56). Ojas, if not depleted
through a poor lifestyle, will give you good immunity, both
physical and mental. This immunity will make you more
resilient to the doshic influences you encounter day by day.

You should also observe the variety of experiences that arise in your mind and body. Note whether they relate to positive or negative aspects of vata, pitta, or kapha. As you do this, you will see how you respond to different qualities in your daily activities. Then you start making choices about the qualities you want to incorporate into your life. You learn to distinguish where your cravings come from: your inner wisdom to balance a dosha or supply a genuine need of your mind or body; or an excess dosha, seeking to increase itself under the principle of "like increases like". Develop your awareness, as your everyday mind will try many tricks to confuse you.

Reviewing your Assessments

Understanding your doshas is an ongoing process, which you will follow automatically as you learn to read the doshas in and around you. Therefore you need to review your assessments to see the doshic patterns in your life.

Try if you can to become aware of any deep feelings that may be subtly influencing your life. These will be very personal and private, but if left unaddressed they may gradually affect your health adversely. Be the observer, and be gentle with yourself as your awareness of these feelings grows.

Use the information from the summary of your assessments (see p. 181) to help you decide which areas of your life you wish to change. Make sure that you are following the correct doshic-pacifying diet (see pp. 154-5).

If you have any current ailments or any doshic imbalance (see p. 63), then you should remove or reduce factors that are increasing the excess dosha(s), or practise acceptance of factors you feel you cannot change (see Chapter Seven). You should follow a lifestyle that will pacify the increased dosha(s). As you deal with your current imbalance, try not to disturb your predominant dosha, if it is different from the increased dosha.

When you have no doshic imbalances, follow a diet and lifestyle that will pacify your predominant dosha(s). This

---

IMPROVING DIGESTION:

- *Correct factors that are disturbing your agni (see p. 76).*
- *Choose a diet suitable for your doshas (see Chapter 6).*
- *Take appropriate exercise (see pp. 96-7).*
- *Eat at regular times and observe the rules of eating (see Chapter 6).*
- *Use herbs and spices that stimulate agni and aid digestion when preparing food and drinks (see pp. 158-65).*
- *Improve your elimination (see pp. 126-7).*

will help you work toward a "better" doshic balance, thereby preventing ailments and illnesses, increasing your vitality, and slowing down the ageing process.

Review possible changes to your lifestyle under these headings: digestion, diet, work, leisure pursuits, exercise, quiet times, morning routine, and responsibility to relationships. Write down your proposals in a positive way rather than a negative way. Let the mind concentrate on the new actions so the old ones will wither through lack of attention. Change should be gradual to be beneficial. Remember that as you change those close to you will have to adjust to the new you.

Make broad statements of intent if you wish to make big changes and then note down the first few small practical steps toward the bigger goal. From your overall list, select two or three small steps to start the process of change. Keep taking further appropriate steps, until you have learned to live and respond to your current experiences, not with habitual reactions, but through aware choices that maintain the natural balance of your doshas.

Seasonal Variations
Whatever your circumstances, you should adjust your lifestyle to allow for seasonal variations (see p. 150).

DIETING

Your body has adapted to your eating patterns. A sudden change in diet can make your body or mind feel deprived. But if the changes are made slowly, both your mind and body have time to adapt.

Permanent changes in weight need to be achieved slowly. Generally, a kapha-pacifying diet will result in weight loss, while a vata-pacifying diet will help you gain weight (see pp. 154-5).

Excess weight may be due to a number of causes, e.g. ama, poor digestion, wrong food combinations, low agni, or overeating (either to satisfy the mind's desire for comfort or the body's need for prana).

Assessment Summary

Use Martin's assessments (see pp. 182-3) to help you summarize your own data. Mark in the related doshas (use the following questions as a guide):-
- What is your constitution or predominant dosha(s)? (See pp. 38-41)
- Are your doshas balanced? (See p. 63)
- Are your predominant dosha(s) or any imbalances increased or pacified by:
  - Your diet
  - Aspects of your work
  - Unresolved emotions
  - Your relationships
  - Your leisure activities
  - Your attitudes
  - Your life events?

VPK and Daily Living

The VPK guidelines below remind you of key points, in addition to the correct diet, for day-to-day living for each constitutional type.

VATA

Have a regular routine • Oil your skin regularly • Take gentle exercise daily • Have plenty of sleep and rest • Keep warm • Nurture your senses

PITTA

Achieve your ambitions without pressurizing yourself • Use constructive criticism rather than confrontation • Take non-competitive exercise daily • Keep cool • Enjoy outdoor activities that challenge you

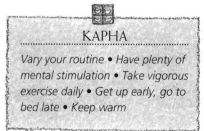

KAPHA

Vary your routine • Have plenty of mental stimulation • Take vigorous exercise daily • Get up early, go to bed late • Keep warm

Caution: If you have any medical condition, dietary or lifestyle changes should be made in consultation with your medical adviser. However, following the correct diet and lifestyle for you will assist any treatments you have.

MARTIN'S ASSESSMENTS

Martin's Ayurvedic profile was described on page 105 and his diet assessed on page 157. Here, his life is related to VPK, and changes and first steps recommended.

Aged 45	*Pitta age*
Constitution	*Pitta*

Ailments

Acid indigestion	*Pitta*
Red spots/blotches	*Pitta*
Lung infections	*Pitta*
Headaches	*Pitta/Vata*

Life Events/Relationships

Aged18 University	*34 Daughter born*
28 Partner in law practice	*37 Son born*
31 Married	*38 Father died*

These all involved changes and increases in vata, but did not have any noticeable effect on his health. At 28, he achieved an ambition, but no definite goals since.

Morning Routine

Erratic, rushing	*Vata*

Work

Responsibilities	*Pitta*
Sedentary	*Kapha*
Travel	*Vata*
Challenging	*Pitta*
Many demands	*Pitta/Vata*
Frustrations	*Pitta*
Interruptions	*Vata*

Leisure

Squash	*Pitta*
Social drinking and eating	*In excess, will increase pitta, kapha*

Digestion

Strong, fast	*Pitta*
Diet	*Pitta*

Attitudes and Emotions

Frustrations	*Pitta*
Deep fear of failure	*Pitta*
Deep fear of emptiness in life	*Vata*

The Summary of Martin's Assessments

Martin's profile reveals a pitta imbalance and a number of pitta influences, though there are also factors which may increase vata. In the past, his health has not been affected by increased vata. But if the vata-increasing factors are not addressed they will be more likely to lead to ailments when he approaches the vata age. Then his body will have less resilience to tolerate further imbalances of doshas due to the prolonged increase of his pitta dosha.

Martin looked closely at his deep inner feelings. In his late teens and twenties, he used his natural pitta energy and the mental abilities manifested from it to gain his legal qualification and successful professional reputation. He developed the habit of achieving, for in addition to his intellectual gifts he had to be very goal-oriented to accomplish his ambition. This habitual way of working (which increases pitta), combined with a deep and private fear of failure, locks him into a pitta-genic lifestyle. Unless he makes changes, such a lifestyle will take him from the early to the later stages of the disease process.

If Martin could reduce his excess pitta energy he would more easily move into the mature stage of his career, reaping broad benefits established by his earlier hard work. He now knows that he should put his positive or natural pitta energy to good use, not only for himself but also for his family and colleagues.

Suggested Changes for Martin to Reduce Pitta

Diet – Pitta-pacifying (see pp. 133-43)

Work – Reduce the demands, frustrations, and interruptions by leading a team to whom he can delegate with confidence, and whose respect he will gain by sharing his experience, by acknowledging their strengths, and by constructively criticizing their weaknesses.

Leisure Pursuits/Exercise – More outdoor activities with his family, e.g. cycling. Some individual sessions with a yoga therapist to establish suitable exercises that he can do each day whether he is home or away.

Morning Routine – Get up early enough to spend half an hour doing yoga or having a quiet time. Eat breakfast with his children.

Responsibility to Relationships — Give uninterrupted time to children/wife without expecting responses or results (since they are unused to this, expectations will limit what could develop). Achieve a better balance between energy and time given to work and family.

Martin's First Steps

Martin accepts that he needs to make changes and apart from the morning routine, the changes he lists are general aims. His first steps are: eating breakfast at the same time as his children; choosing foods more carefully when eating out; becoming aware of when he is impatient or critical with his personal assistant; reflecting on more appropriate ways of responding; and making an appointment with a yoga therapist.

SEEKING ADVICE

If you feel unsure about taking steps to change your lifestyle and would like Ayurvedic advice, then you can seek either an Ayurvedic physician or practitioner. The former has had extensive and rigorous training: a degree in Ayurvedic Medicine and Surgery, which takes five years to complete, is followed by a period of supervised practical experience – similar to the internship of newly graduated Western doctors.

In 1980, Dr. Robert Svoboda (who wrote the foreword to this book) became the first Westerner to graduate from a recognized university or college with such a degree. He is one of a very few fully trained Ayurvedic physicians practising in the West. This situation may slowly change. In India, more Ayurveda students than ever are receiving training and more Ayurvedic clinics are catering for Westerners.

Currently, in the West, Ayurveda is used primarily for prevention and alleviation of digestive disorders. Increasing numbers of Westerners are seeking training in its principles and practice. They may become Ayurvedic practitioners, not physicians. Those sufficiently trained already can offer guidance on panchakarma (see p. 186), herbs, diet, and lifestyle. Some Western health-care practitioners and alternative therapists are receiving instruction in Ayurveda to complement their professional expertise. This will enable them to make individual assessments, be more effective in selecting treatments, and offer dietary and lifestyle advice using Ayurvedic principles.

Finding an Ayurvedic physician or practitioner can be difficult. Not only are they few and far between at present, but also standards may vary. However, this will change, too. Standards of training for different levels of practitioners and registers of practitioners are yet to be established. Consequently, when you try to find a competent Ayurvedic physician or practitioner, use your common sense and be guided by your inner wisdom – do not let your good judgment be clouded by a desperate desire to find help.

Assessing Ill Health

Good powers of observation and a deep understanding of
the body enable Ayurvedic physicians to read information
about health and illness from small signs. They then build a
complete picture of a patient's doshic balance or imbalance.
In making an assessment, the physician needs to ascertain
which doshas, tissues, channels, and organs are affected,
and will need to discover your constitution, the strength of
your agni and your strength to undertake treatment.
Physicians ask questions to confirm assessments they make
by reading the pulse or observing the tongue, iris, face,
skin, urine, and stools.

Ayurvedic Treatments

The object of treatment in Ayurveda is to restore the
patient's natural balance of the doshas by pacification, thus
removing the cause of the illness as well as the symptoms.
When the doshic balance is restored, the tissues weakened
by the illness need to be rejuvenated. The effectiveness of
the treatment will depend on many factors including your
physical and mental strength to overcome the illness, the
length of time you have suffered from it, your age, your
diligence in following the advice, and the accuracy of the
advice. The longer you have had an illness, the longer and
harder it is to restore your doshic balance. It is also harder
to restore the doshic balance and rejuvenate the tissues
completely when you are in the vata age since your metabolism is naturally slowing down.

Herbs, panchakarma (see p. 186) and shirodhara (see
right) are the principal treatments used in Ayurveda in the
West, but many other treatments now available in the West
as complementary therapies have been used within
Ayurveda for thousands of years. These include massage,
marma point manipulation (similar to acupressure), colour
and gem therapy, essences and potencised remedies, music
and chanting, meditation, yoga, and balancing nadi energy
(on which polarity therapy is based).

SHIRODHARA

*Shirodhara is the con-
tinuous flow of warm
oil over the forehead. It
can give a very deep
state of relaxation, and
helps release deep
unresolved emotions. It
is very soothing for an
agitated mind.
Shirodhara may also be
given as part of a pan-
chakarma programme.*

The Use of Herbs

In Ayurveda, herbs are often used for pacification (and the rejuvenation that follows) and the general maintenance of health. A vast range of herbs is available and their effectiveness is due to detailed knowledge of their special actions, or prabhav (see p. 53) and correctly matching these to the doshas, tissues, and agni.

Ayurveda understands herbs in terms of their qualities and their effects in the body and on the doshas. Thus it is concerned with the overall strengthening or diminishing action in the body not the "active" ingredient of each herb. In Ayurveda, a medicine should do its job in the body and leave without side effects. Although many Ayurvedic herbal formulae are available as general tonics, individual treatments are finely tuned to the patient's constitution and specific circumstances as well as the doshas and tissues involved.

Panchakarma

If you have the physical strength, the physician may suggest purification in the form of panchakarma. This deep cleansing process, which is unique to Ayurveda, enables the body to release excess doshas and toxins from its cells, gather them in the gastro-intestinal tract, and expel them. Panchakarma means five actions. These are therapeutic vomiting to remove excess kapha, therapeutic purgation to remove excess pitta, therapeutic enema to remove excess vata, nasal administration in cases of diseases of the head, ` and neck and blood-letting in cases of blood disorders.

The body has to be properly prepared for a number of days. This involves deep, generous oil massage followed by steam treatment. The steam helps the oil penetrate the skin as well as releasing surface toxins. Herbs may be used with the oil or steam. When the oil has penetrated deeply and the body is fully prepared, the appropriate "action" is taken. Each panchakarma programme is individually tailored to the patient.

Pulse Diagnosis

Some Ayurvedic physicians rely solely on pulse diagnosis to determine health. Usually taken at the radial arteries in the wrist, it is a skill that requires great sensitivity, clarity, and dedication to acquire. In the hands of an expert, it is very accurate, though you may find it disconcerting to have such a short consultation.

PACIFICATION

This involves "burning" ama, enkindling agni, and removing excess doshas, using herbs, fasting under supervision, exercise, and pranayama.

Caution: *Panchakarma is very powerful and should be carried out by an experienced practitioner.*

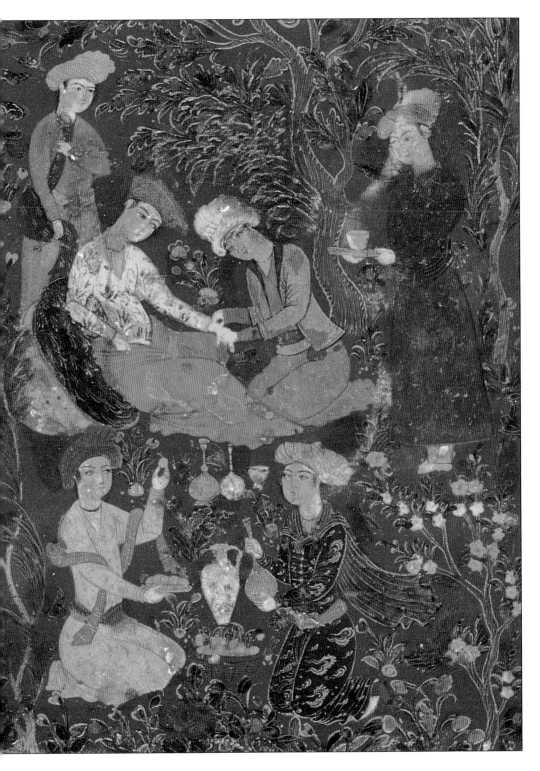

INDEX